# Homegrown
# Remedies

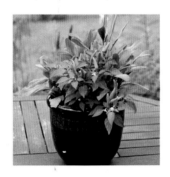

D1737596

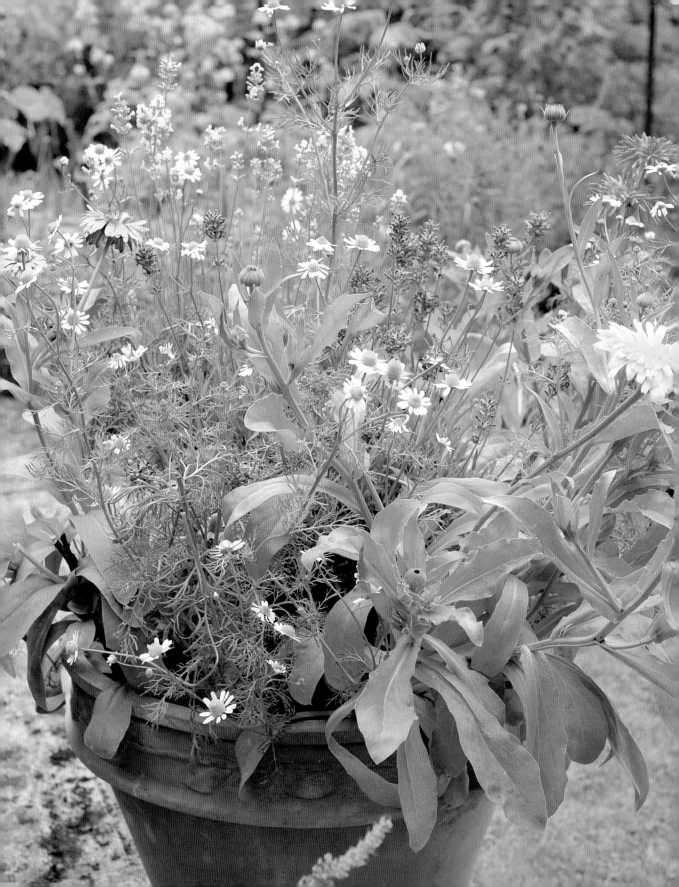

# Homegrown
# Remedies

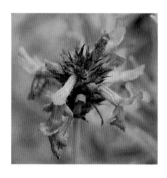

## Anne McIntyre

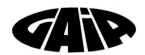

First published in Great Britain in 2011 by
Gaia, a division of Octopus Publishing Group Ltd
Endeavour House
189 Shaftesbury Avenue
London
WC2H 8JY
www.octopusbooksusa.com

Distributed in the USA and Canada for Octopus Books USA
c/o Hachette Book Group USA
237 Park Avenue
New York, NY 10017

Copyright © Octopus Publishing Group Ltd 2011
Text copyright © Anne McIntyre 2011

All rights reserved. No part of this work may be reproduced or utilized in any form or by any
means, electronic or mechanical, including photocopying, recording or by any information
storage and retrieval system, without the prior written permission of the publisher.

Anne McIntyre asserts the moral right to be identified as the author of this book.

ISBN 978-1-84601-386-7

A CIP catalogue record for this book is available from the British Library.

Printed and bound in China

10 9 8 7 6 5 4 3 2 1

This book contains the opinions and ideas of the author. It is intended to provide helpful and
informative material on the subjects addressed in this book and is sold with the understanding
that the author and publisher are not engaged in rendering any kind of personal professional
services in this book. The author and publisher disclaim all responsibility for any liability, loss or
risk, personal or otherwise, that is incurred as a consequence, directly or indirectly, of the use
and application of any of the contents of this book.

All reasonable care has been taken in the preparation of this book, but the information it contains
is not meant to take the place of medical care under the direct supervision of a doctor. Before
making any changes in your health regime, always consult a doctor. While all the remedies
detailed in this book are completely safe if made correctly, you must seek professional advice if
you are in any doubt about any medical condition. Any application of the ideas and information
contained in this book is at the reader's sole discretion and risk.

# Contents

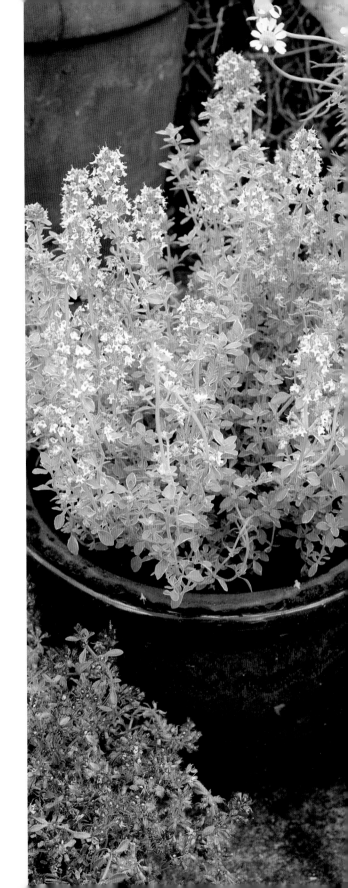

# Introduction

## How to use herbs for healing

Gardening is one of the best kinds of preventative medicine; good for all manner of ills. If you love gardening, as I do, you will probably have experienced that sense of joy derived from hours spent nurturing plants and seeing them develop in shape, form and colour. For many people, the garden is their sanctuary, a place of peace and refreshment, away from the stress of everyday life. Even if you do not have space for a garden, you can still create form and beauty, not forgetting wonderful scents, from herbs grown in pots and containers, whether inside or out. When you grow herbs you will have the reward of harvesting those herbs and using them to enhance your health and wellbeing.

Growing herbs is an excellent way to get to know plants that are not only beautiful and evocatively scented but also remarkable medicines. Herbs are a very real part of everyday life; they enliven diet and cuisine, provide valuable ingredients for beauty products, cosmetics, toothpastes, body creams and lotions and also play an important part in health care. Many common herbs used by herbalists to help and cure everyday ailments can be found in your kitchen, on your patio or in the garden, in nearby parks, fields and hedgerows, and you can prepare them at home, simply and quickly. A sage gargle, for example, makes an effective cure for sore throats; hot mint and honey drinks ease colds and catarrh; vinegar soothes wasp stings and dock leaves rubbed on to nettle stings provide ready relief. Sowing herb seeds and watching them grow or raising smaller plants, caring for them, then snipping off leaves and flowers to add to tasty recipes – foods, tisanes, tinctures, massage oils and body creams – can bring you into a closer relationship with your health and an awareness of the amazing tools you have around you to treat common ailments. Your garden, patio or window sill can be your instant medicine cabinet, enabling you to treat a wide range of everyday coughs and colds, catarrh, stomach aches, headaches and general aches and pains. This means that you can cut down the visits to your doctor and the need to use powerful medicines for minor, self-limiting illnesses. It makes ecological and economical sense and it's surprisingly easy to do.

### A little bit of history

The relationship between humans and plants has always been fundamental. For millennia we relied on plants for food, clothing, shelter and fuel, and even for protection against the invisible and incomprehensible – the powers of darkness, thunder and the 'evil eye', which our ancestors believed were responsible for illness of body or soul. Plants are the source of all the foods we enjoy and the oxygen we breathe, and so it is hardly surprising that for thousands of years they also provided us with medicines for treating almost every ailment. Medicinal herbs have been

*You can grow one plant per pot, or an assortment of different herbs together in a larger pot, to create a medley of colour and scents.*

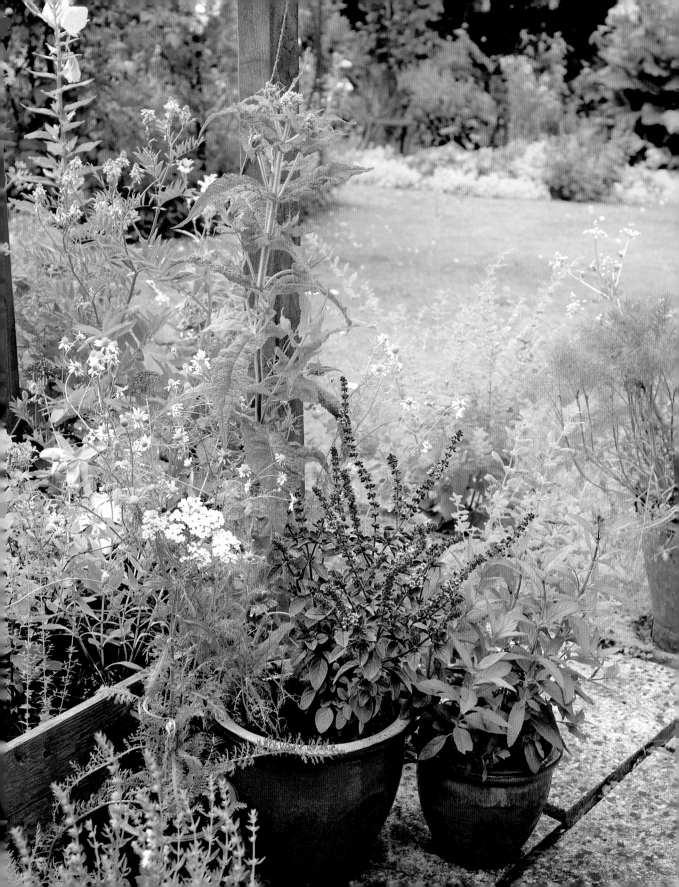

used in cultures all over the world in their different healing systems, for as far back as records go. We know that herbs have been used for healing and for their symbolic significance right from Neanderthal times. In 1963 archeologists found several herbs buried in a grave, made 60,000 years ago, in a cave in Iraq. As far back as 3,000 BC schools of herbal medicine existed in Egypt, China, Assyria and India. Some of the earliest written evidence comes from Chinese treatises attributed to the Yellow Emperor around 2,500 BC called the *Pen T'sao*. Other written records date from the time of the Ancient Egyptians, who inscribed recipes for herbal mixtures on clay tablets and papyrus.

In ancient systems of healing herbs were revered for their success in treating not only physical illnesses, but also imbalances in the realm of emotion, mind and spirit. Their mythologies and religions incorporated the use of plants, often in rituals, and herbs were used for problems ranging from broken legs to unfulfilled dreams and soul loss. Flowers and herbs had symbolic meaning, which was used in China, Egypt and India, for example, as a form of communication. We can also see this in Elizabethan England in Shakespeare's plays, when most of the audiences would have been familiar with his plant references and their hidden meanings.

Our ancestors' knowledge and insight into the successful use of indigenous plants as medicines for body, mind and spirit has survived through generations to give us a rich heritage of accumulated knowledge backed by thousands of years of practical experience. We are lucky to be able to benefit from this wisdom and experience. There is a wealth of information available about the amazing healing world of herbs that you can

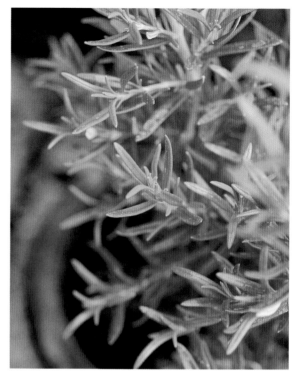

*Rosemary one of the most important and versatile of the healing herbs available for our use.*

dip into and a body of professional herbalists available, should you need further help or advice.

Tending your herb garden may stimulate your curiosity and entice you to learn more about these incredible plants. You may be surprised to discover how many common garden plants, wild flowers or even nuisance 'weeds' are valuable herbal remedies and have potent therapeutic compounds. Poppies, violets, plantains, pansies, self-heal, roses, dandelions and even couch grass spring instantly to mind. Apparently simple herbs that will grow easily in most soils have warranted much time and money invested in research as potential cures to illnesses such as viral infection, immune deficiency, depression, malaria, peptic ulcers and many acute and degenerative, as well as stress-related, disorders. Echinacea, St John's wort, aloe vera, holy basil and gotu kola are examples of such valuable herbs. Your medicinal garden can include healing plants from all over the world that will grow in a temperate climate. Among these are: Indian herbs gotu kola, lemon grass, coriander, holy basil, cumin and fenugreek, Chinese remedies codonopsis, Baikal skullcap and self-heal, or native American medicines such as boneset, California poppy, cayenne, skullcap and echinacea.

## Returning to our roots

With the wide availability of modern drugs we may have forgotten our simple, readily available herbal remedies, but they are now beginning to have their place in the sun again. Traditional plant remedies provide about 85 per cent of the world's medicines and so make a significant contribution to healthcare worldwide. With their myriad therapeutic actions they can provide safe, effective and time-proven alternatives to orthodox drugs. They make excellent preventive medicines and can enhance general wellbeing alongside a healthy diet and lifestyle. They can also bring symptomatic relief (for example for first aid and minor infections), helping us to avoid the use of drugs, such as antibiotics, when they are unnecessary.

Research into the medicinal value of herbs and foods is increasing worldwide as scientists continue their search for new 'cures' for problems such as heart disease, degenerative disease and cancer. Studies have identified the chemically active ingredients in many herbs, explaining their ancient use as medicines. Folk remedies such as celery seed for arthritis, garlic for the heart and blood pressure, thyme for infections and cayenne pepper for pain relief have been found to have scientific merit. This is unsurprising when you consider that many major medical discoveries and potent medicines, used in the highly scientific approach to modern medicine, originate in nature – penicillin from bread mould, digoxin from foxglove and aspirin from willow. So if you want to understand more about how the simple herbs you grow in pots and containers work, there is plenty of material available. You can use your home-grown remedies, priding yourself in the fact that they are inexpensive, practical, readily available and – most importantly – they work.

## How do herbs work?

Herbs are made up of natural constituents that have an inherent compatibility with our bodies. We cannot directly assimilate many of the substances our bodies need to grow to maintain our health and to heal us when we are ill. Plants process these substances for us, making them accessible to the body. Through photosynthesis plants manufacture carbohydrates and give off oxygen, while taking up minerals and trace elements through their roots. This creates metabolic pathways that provide building blocks for the production of compounds that can easily be utilized in the body. In medicinal plants these include minerals, vitamins and trace elements, the raw materials we need for recovery, as well as a vast assortment of other medicinal substances such as volatile oils, bitters, tannins and alkaloids, which have affinities for particular organs and systems and specific therapeutic actions in the body.

Herbs are very much like foods and the dividing line between them is very thin. A herbal remedy is, by definition, any plant which has a therapeutic action and this includes most of the fruit and vegetable kingdom. Celery seeds and celery have a cleansing, antiseptic effect through the whole of the urinary tract and are widely used for arthritis; oats are a wonderful tonic to the nervous system, while raspberries have long been used for throat and chest problems.

We have always eaten plants and so the human body has adapted over millennia to respond to plant medicines in a way that it cannot possibly respond to powerful synthetic drugs. This means that there is less risk of side effects when using herbs as medicines. The substances that plants contain are very similar in chemical make-up to those that form the human body.

### What can herbs do?
Apart from the huge benefit to your wellbeing brought about by the happy hours spent tending them, herbs themselves have diverse medicinal actions. They contain a huge range of therapeutic substances and have a variety of different actions, related to the combined effect of these components. These include tannins, volatile oils, mucilage, alkaloids, glycosides, saponins, flavonoids and bitters. They are found in varying proportions in different parts of the plant. Sometimes we use the roots, at other times the leaves, flowers, berries or bark. In some instances we use many different parts of the plant, each one for a different therapeutic effect. For example, mullein is a herb found wild, often as a garden weed. The leaves, flowers, roots and fruit can all be used. The flowers and leaves can be made into ointment and used externally for haemorrhoids, while a flower infusion can be used to relieve pain, induce sleep and as a laxative. A hot mullein leaf poultice will help relieve mastitis, while the root and leaves have

*Opposite A combination of yarrow and chamomile is a good remedy for fevers and infections.*

been used in infusion and decoction for colds, coughs, asthma, hay fever, glandular swellings, rheumatism and diarrhoea.

Herbs also differ in their remedial action, depending on how the plant is prepared and taken. Sage is a good example: the essential oil in its leaves, which lend the herb its characteristic odour, is antiseptic and fungicidal. Sage leaves also contain astringent tannin and a bitter compound called picrosalvine. The disinfectant action of sage tea is due to the combined effect of these components and is best used in gargles for sore throats and mouthwashes for inflamed gums.

When the tea is swallowed, other qualities of the plant become apparent. Sage can help prevent night sweats and abate the flow of breast milk when mothers are weaning their babies. The volatile oil in sage contains a substance called thujone. If sage tea is drunk on a regular basis over a long period of time or in large amounts it can bring on menstrual flow, and for this reason it should not be taken in pregnancy. However, it can be helpful if a baby is overdue, when it may be recommended to stimulate contractions.

### Your container herb garden
The 40 pots described in this book and the recipes suggested for treating a range of common ailments are designed to give you an idea of the potential uses of the herbs at your fingertips. By growing the herbs and trying out the recipes you will gain practical experience of how easy it is to use your container garden as an instant source of medicines. If you are treating a

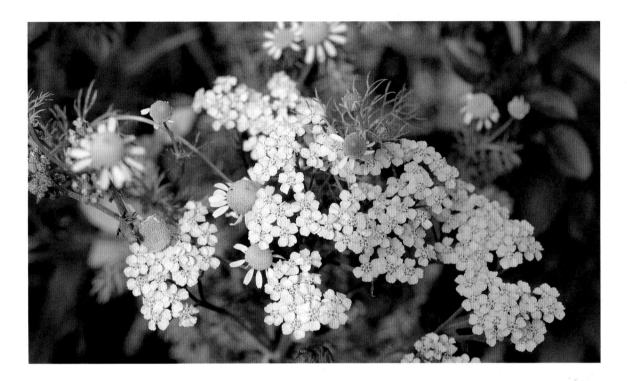

chronic problem, such as irritable bowel syndrome or arthritis, you may need to supplement the herbs you grow with other herbs bought in, either in dried or tincture form. You can also plant up other containers, should you wish, for other ailments. By referring to the herb and plant directory at the end of the book (see page 118), you will be able to find out which herbs best suit your particular needs and design a container just for you.

When treating common ailments at home it is always important to exercise caution. You need to be sure what plants you are using by clearly labelling them. If you buy them in pots, already grown, they need to come from a reputable supplier and also be clearly labelled. If acute symptoms do not clear within a few days, and chronic symptoms do not improve within three to four weeks, see your doctor.

By creating a medicinal, or apothecary's, garden among your pots you will be following in the footsteps of many an eminent herbalist and herb gardener of the past, maintaining the continuity of herb gardening through history.

Plants that have been grown by priests, physicians and apothecaries down the millennia are little changed today – cowslips, periwinkles, violets and roses are as popular as inhabitants of herb gardens today as they were over 1,000 years ago in medieval monastery gardens.

Such plants and gardens connect us to all the men and women who gardened, cooked and healed with them, just as we do now. They represent a living history, connecting us to a time when plants were valued not only for their earthly gifts but also for their benefits in the realm of the spirit.

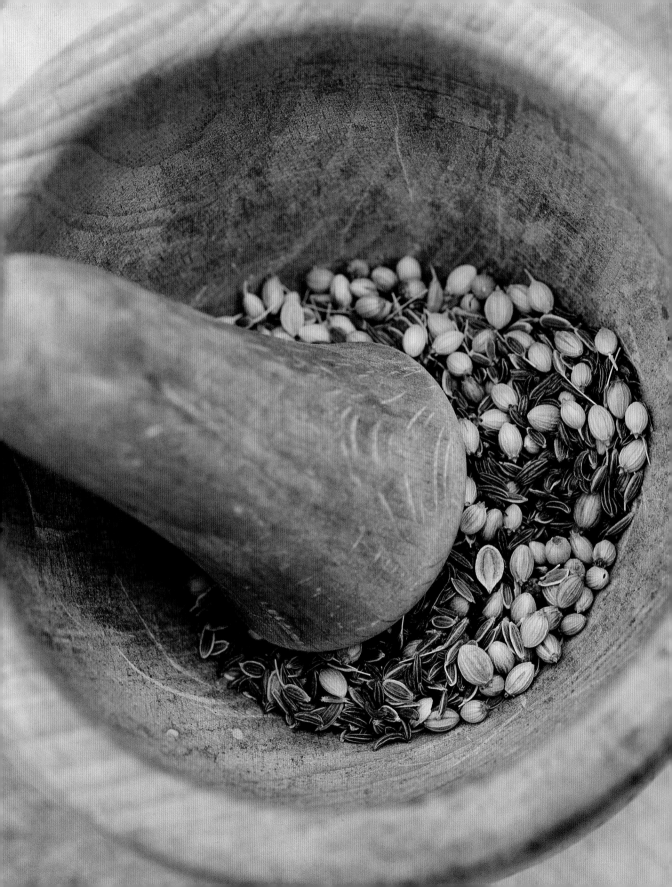

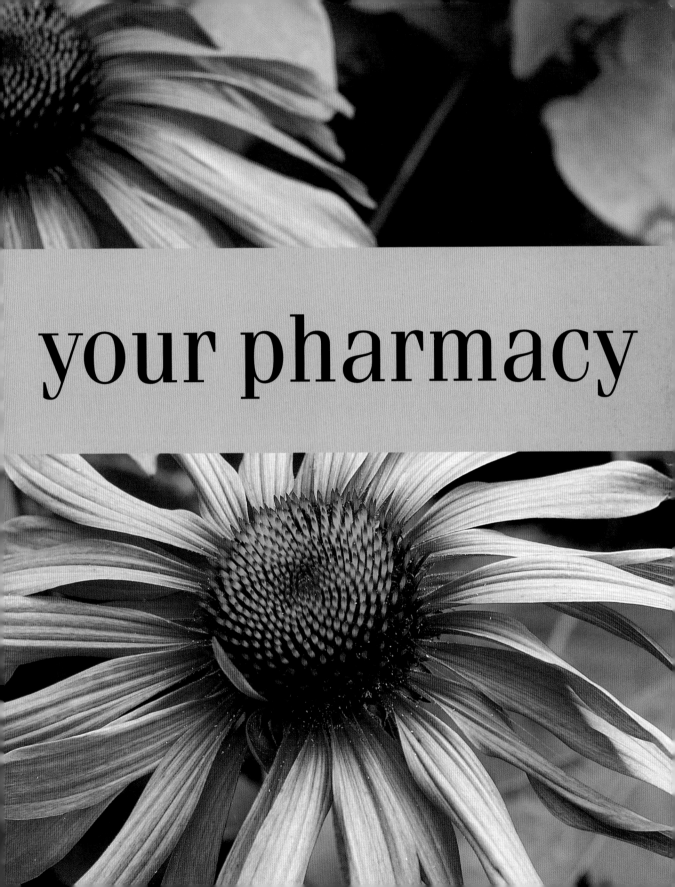

# your pharmacy

# How to use herbs

## Healing at your fingertips

Making herbal remedies from the herbs you have grown in pots can be fun, easy and economical. It is best to pick your herbs first thing in the morning so that they're as fresh as possible. Choose the healthiest-looking parts of the plant, wash them under cold water, remove soil and old leaves and pat them dry.

There are many ways you can take herbs, to benefit from their healing actions. The easiest way is in food and drink, which many people do by taking culinary herbs and herbal teas, often without realizing their medicinal action.

Salads with basil, coriander leaves, rocket and parsley, vinaigrette with garlic, fish with dill or sorrel, new potatoes with fresh mint, casseroles with bay leaves and pizza with oregano are all very familiar. Once your food is absorbed, the nutrients and therapeutic constituents of the herbs enter the bloodstream and then circulate around the body. Your favourite culinary herbs all contain volatile oils that lend their wonderful flavours and scents. These oils have anti-microbial properties, helping to fight off a wide variety of infections. You can also prepare a choice of different herbal preparations including tinctures, syrups, capsules and honeys. Another way is to make preparations to apply to the skin, which is very absorbent and covers a large surface area. Tiny capillaries take the medicinal compounds in the herbs into the bloodstream and to the body. You can use infusions as hand and foot baths, massage oils into the skin, apply

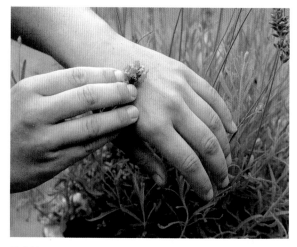

*Rubbing lavender flowers directly on to the skin can relieve burns and insect bites.*

tincture-based rubbing lotions and ointments, creams, compresses and poultices. In addition, fresh herbs can be applied directly, such as aloe vera gel to soothe a sting or lavender flowers to staunch bleeding from minor cuts and abrasions and to relieve minor burns.

The conjunctiva of the eye will also absorb herbal extracts. A plantain or chamomile eyebath will relieve sore and inflamed eyes. The nose and the nerve endings in the eye can provide another therapeutic pathway utilized by aromatherapists. When we use a hot tea or herbal oil as an inhalation, the messages from the herbs are carried directly to the brain and are also taken into the lungs where they are absorbed with oxygen into the bloodstream and circulated throughout the body.

## Nutrients found in our favourite herbs

### VITAMINS

| | |
|---|---|
| **Vitamin A** | Dandelion ◆ gotu kola ◆ fenugreek ◆ rocket ◆ plantain ◆ cayenne ◆ basil ◆ dill ◆ peppermint ◆ rosemary ◆ parsley ◆ sage ◆ coriander |
| **Vitamin B** | Fenugreek ◆ parsley ◆ peppermint ◆ sage ◆ coriander ◆ garlic ◆ dandelion |
| **Vitamin C** | Echinacea ◆ garlic ◆ peppermint ◆ rosehips ◆ sorrel ◆ dandelion ◆ fenugreek ◆ rocket ◆ dill ◆ rosemary ◆ basil ◆ parsley ◆ sage ◆ coriander ◆ caraway ◆ oregano |
| **Vitamin D** | Dandelion ◆ rosehips |
| **Vitamin E** | Dandelion ◆ skullcap ◆ parsley ◆ sage |
| **Vitamin K** | Gotu kola ◆ basil ◆ parsley ◆ sage ◆ coriander ◆ dandelion |
| **Niacin** | Feverfew ◆ fenugreek ◆ parsley ◆ peppermint |
| **Vitamin P** | Cayenne |

### MINERALS

| | |
|---|---|
| **Calcium** | Aloe vera ◆ cayenne pepper ◆ chamomile ◆ fennel ◆ marshmallow ◆ sage ◆ dill ◆ peppermint ◆ rosemary ◆ parsley ◆ caraway ◆ garlic ◆ oregano ◆ coriander ◆ dandelion |
| **Cobalt** | Dandelion ◆ parsley ◆ cayenne pepper ◆ echinacea root |
| **Iron** | Nettles ◆ peppermint ◆ rosemary ◆ skullcap ◆ dill ◆ parsley ◆ sage ◆ coriander ◆ caraway ◆ garlic ◆ oregano ◆ dandelion |
| **Magnesium** | Gotu kola ◆ rosemary ◆ wood betony ◆ basil ◆ dill ◆ peppermint ◆ parsley ◆ sage ◆ caraway ◆ oregano ◆ coriander ◆ dandelion, |
| **Manganese** | Basil ◆ dill ◆ rosemary ◆ peppermint ◆ sage ◆ coriander ◆ caraway ◆ garlic ◆ oregano ◆ dandelion |
| **Potassium** | Aloe vera ◆ dandelion ◆ cayenne ◆ fennel ◆ parsley ◆ rosehips ◆ wild celery ◆ dill ◆ rosemary ◆ peppermint ◆ oregano |
| **Zinc** | Chamomile ◆ skullcap ◆ dandelion ◆ marshmallow ◆ rosemary ◆ peppermint ◆ sage ◆ caraway ◆ garlic ◆ coriander |
| **Chromium** | Nettles |
| **Copper** | Skullcap ◆ sage ◆ dill ◆ rosemary ◆ peppermint ◆ garlic ◆ coriander |
| **Selenium** | Garlic ◆ coriander |

# Internal preparations

## Herbs you can take

### Infusions

Infusions, or teas, are the easiest and most common way to prepare leaves, stems and flowers – using the same method as you would to make a normal cup of tea. The hot water extracts herb constituents if you leave it to steep. You can use a favourite teapot, a cafetière, a stainless-steel infuser ball or teabags. The usual ratio is 25 g (1 oz) of dried herb per 600 ml (1 pint) of water or a teaspoon of dried herb per cupful of water. If you are using fresh herbs, double the quantity.

When making tea in a pot, place the herbs in the warmed pot and pour over boiling water. Cover immediately to prevent volatile oils escaping. Leave to infuse for 10 to 15 minutes and strain. Drink immediately or store it in the fridge for up to two days.

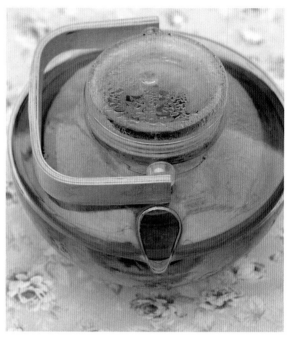

*Herbs need to be infused, preferably in a tea pot, for 10–15 minutes before drinking.*

The therapeutic components of some of the more soothing herbs may be destroyed by high temperatures and, therefore, need to be prepared as cold infusions. These include herbs that have a high proportion of mucilage such as marshmallow, plantain and comfrey leaf. The method and dosage is the same, but they are covered with cold water and left to infuse for 10 to 12 hours.

**Dosage:** You can take infusions three times a day for chronic symptoms and up to six times daily (up to 200 ml/a cupful at a time) for acute problems such as sore throats, flu and chest

infections. Many people are accustomed to sweet-tasting foods and medicines and find it hard to adjust to the unfamiliar flavours of some herbs. Although bitters need to be tasted to be effective, the taste can be hard to accept. However, it is possible to combine several herbs in an infusion to allow pleasant-tasting herbs, such as peppermint, fennel, lemon balm and lavender, to mask the flavour of less palatable herbs, while not reducing their effect. Licorice and fennel are superb herbs for adding flavour. You can also sweeten infusions with honey. Infusions are usually taken warm to hot, particularly when treating fevers, colds and catarrh. They are taken lukewarm to cold for problems associated with the kidneys and urinary tract, such as kidney infections, cystitis, urethritis and bed-wetting.

### Decoctions

The hard woody parts of plants have tough cell walls and need high temperatures to break them down before their constituents can be extracted by the water. Bark, seeds, roots, rhizomes and nuts all need to be prepared as decoctions. Break the herb into small pieces with a pestle and mortar or smash them with a hammer; their constituents will be more accessible to water.

Use the same ratio of herbs to water as you do for an infusion, but add a little more water to compensate for loss during boiling. Place herbs in a saucepan and cover with water. Bring to the boil, cover and simmer for 10 to 15 minutes. Strain and drink as an infusion.

### Tinctures

Tinctures are concentrated herbal extracts that utilize a mixture of water and alcohol or glycerol to extract plant constituents and act as a preservative. There is a correct ratio of water and alcohol to plant matter for each herb, depending on the constituents requiring extraction. It can range from 25 per cent alcohol for simple glycosides and tannins to 90 per cent for resins and gums such as those in marigold flowers. When making tinctures you can easily use neat vodka, brandy or gin, which are about 45 per cent alcohol and these will act as good extractives and preservatives.

You can use fresh or dried, finely chopped or powdered herbs. Place the herb in a large jar

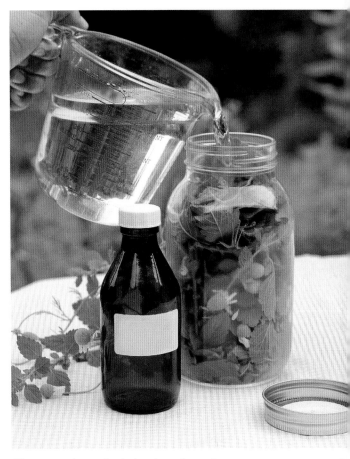

*Place your chosen herbs in a large jar and pour on a glycerol and alcohol mix to make a glycerite.*

and pour over the alcohol or alcohol mixture. If you use dried herbs, the ratio is one part of herbs per five parts of liquid; fresh herbs are used in a ratio of one part herb to two parts liquid. For example, to make 1 litre (1¾ pint) of chamomile tincture, take 200 g (7 oz) of dried flowers and pour over 1 litre (1¾ pint) of fluid. Chamomile requires a 45 per cent alcohol solution and brandy or vodka would be acceptable. Pour the fluid over the herb, place an airtight lid on the jar and leave to macerate away from direct sunlight for at least two weeks. Shake the jar once a day. Then squeeze the mixture through a press to extract maximum fluid. Throw the herb away, transfer the tincture to a dark bottle and store in a cool place.

You can use neat cider vinegar to prepare tinctures as the acetic acid acts as a solvent and preservative. Raspberry vinegar, for example, is a traditional remedy for coughs and sore throats. You can also use glycerol. Glycerol-based tinctures have a sweet taste, which makes them a good medium for children's medicines.

Pour equal parts of water and glycerol over the herbs, using the same proportion of herb to liquid as for alcohol tinctures. Eighty per cent glycerol is needed for more watery fresh herbs such as marshmallow and coltsfoot, to prevent deterioration. Peppermint, lemon balm,

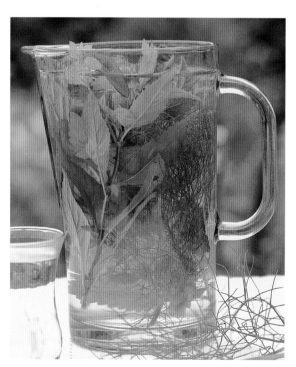

*Transform your drinking water by infusing aromatic herbs in a jug of water for a few hours.*

*Opposite When making a tincture place the herbs in a glass jar and pour over a mixture of alcohol and water.*

lavender, rose, basil, elderflower and catmint are ideal for this method. If you want to ensure that your glycerol tincture will not deteriorate you can use 80 per cent glycerol and 20 per cent alcohol instead of water.

As tinctures are concentrated; you need only take small amounts regularly through the day. The dose will vary from five to ten drops to a teaspoon, in a little warm water, fruit juice or herbal tea, three to six times daily, depending on whether the condition is chronic or acute.

Tinctures can also be added to bath water, mixed with water to make compresses, mouthwashes or gargles, or stirred into a base to make ointments or creams. Tinctures require more preparation, but are easy to store, do not deteriorate in cold or damp conditions, take up relatively little space and keep almost indefinitely, although they are best used within two years.

## Syrups

Herbal syrups are designed to make herbal preparations more palatable, so that they can be taken by children and sensitive adults. Bitter herbs such as dandelion, rosemary, vervain and motherwort are particularly suited. Expectorant herbs for coughs, asthma and chest infections such as thyme, hyssop and basil are often prepared as syrups, particularly when honey is used. Syrups can also be added to other preparations to mask unpleasant tastes.

You can make a syrup in different ways. When using a tincture, pour 600 ml (1 pint) of boiling

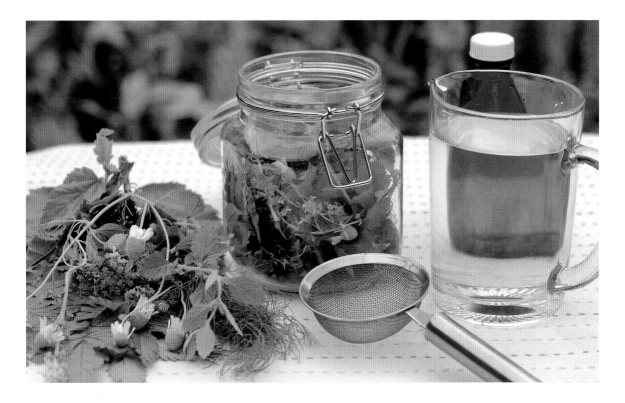

water over 1.25 kg (2½ lb) of soft brown sugar in a pan and stir over gentle heat until all sugar has dissolved and the solution comes to the boil. Remove from the heat and cool. Choose the herbal tincture you'd like to use for your syrup and add it in the ratio of one part tincture to three parts syrup. Store the syrup in sterilized dark glass bottles with cork stoppers, labelled clearly, and it will keep for up to two years.

Alternatively use an infusion or decoction. Make a double-strength infusion/decoction of your chosen herb, leave it to infuse overnight then strain it into a jug and press residual water from the herb before discarding. Mix 500 g (1 lb) sugar into 600 ml (1 pint) of the infusion/decoction in a pan and heat it until the sugar has dissolved and the mixture has started to thicken, stirring frequently. If desired, add five per cent of the same tincure to preserve the syrup. Store in sterilized, dark bottles, clearly labelled, and keep in a cool place, preferably the fridge, for a maximum of six months.

You can also use honey to make a syrup. Using an infusion or decoction of the herb of your choice, strain it and then weigh it and add it to a quarter of its weight in honey. Heat the liquid slowly and stir it until it begins to thicken, skimming off scum. Store in clearly labelled, sterilized bottles. It is better to use a cork stopper because syrups can ferment and may blow the stopper out. Don't use bottles with screw tops – they could explode!

**Dosage:** one dessertspoonful three or four times a day for chronic symptoms and double the amount for acute problems.

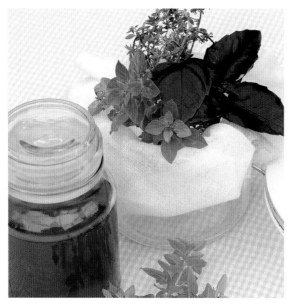

*The sweet taste of honey brings out the great flavours of aromatic herbs.*

## Honey

Honey is a good medium for herbal preparations as the sweet taste brings out the aromatic flavours of the herbs and also extracts and preserves their therapeutic components. It actually increases their preservation and so extends shelf life. Honey is hydroscopic, meaning that it absorbs the water-soluble constituents and volatile oils in herbs. It has antibacterial, expectorant and healing properties, so herbal honeys are good for acute infections, sore throats, coughs, chest infections, asthma, and externally to heal or soothe skin problems such as cuts and grazes, burns and varicose ulcers. It makes an excellent medium for antimicrobial herbs such as garlic, thyme, hyssop, oregano and rosemary. It is also highly nutritive, high in easily digestible sugars, and is energy-giving and enhances the immune system. It contains pollen that is rich in protein, vitamins, minerals and fatty acids and is helpful in the treatment of

allergies and asthma, and propolis, which is a powerful antimicrobial. Thyme honey from Greece is renowned for its health-giving properties, as is Manuka honey from New Zealand, which is often used as an antibacterial.

The simplest, most immediate, way to use honey is to mix freshly chopped or dried, powdered herbs in a teaspoon of good organic honey and given on a spoon three to six times a day. You can also prepare herbs in honey to preserve them for longer in the following way:

Place the herbs, coarsely chopped, in a clean, sterilized jar. You can use a reusable teabag or tie the herbs into a piece of muslin. Cover them with honey and stir well. Close with an airtight lid, label clearly and leave to macerate for at least four weeks and remove the herbs. Store in a cool, dark place, preferably the fridge.

A faster method involves using a double boiler. Add one to two cups of the chopped herb directly to two cups of honey, or use a reusable teabag or muslin bag to contain the herbs. Heat the mixture in a double boiler for four to five hours and then strain it or remove the teabag and pour into a jar. Store as above. If you want a more delicately flavored honey, you can also use aromatic flowers or leaves of thyme, hyssop, lavender, roses or lemon balm. For a stronger flavour, try cayenne pepper.

To make garlic honey use six to eight cloves of garlic to one cup of raw, organic honey. Put the honey and peeled garlic cloves in a heavy-bottomed saucepan and heat gently over medium-low heat until it boils. Remove from the heat and when cool, pour into a clean, sterilized jar and seal with a lid. Keep in a cool place, out

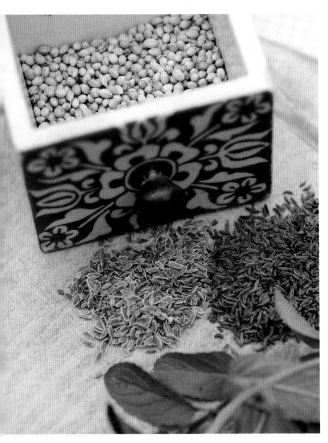

*A spicy oxymel, as used in times gone by, can make an energizing start to the day.*

of sunlight, and use as needed. Dosage is one tablespoonful of herbal honey in a little hot water or from a spoon. Do not give it to children who are under the age of one, due to risk of botulinus in raw sugar.

You can also make sweets and throat lozenges by rolling powdered herbs in honey to make a paste, which can be rolled into balls and then again in the powder to prevent stickiness for handling and storing. Store them in a tightly fitting tin. Honey and herbs combined are a delicious way to take herbs and are excellent for children. These are also known as 'electuaries'.

## Oxymels

An oxymel is a combination of infused cider vinegar and honey, the use of which originated in the Middle East and was brought to England after the Crusades.

Apparently knights and their ladies drank hot oxymels for breakfast as a stimulating way to start the day. Both the honey and the vinegar act as extractives and preservatives for the herbs and make a pleasant-tasting preparation.

If you want to have a go at making an oxymel yourself, place 50 ml (2 fl oz) of a herbal vinegar and 100 g (4 oz) of honey into a heavy-bottomed saucepan. Heat slowly and leave it alone until the mixture has reduced by one-third to 100 ml (4 fl oz). Then strain the mixture, allow it to cool thoroughly, and transfer it to sterilized bottles with cork stoppers. Label them clearly.

**Dosage:** Take two teaspoonfuls between three and six times daily.

## Elixirs

Honey can also be combined with brandy to make elixirs, which are an easy and delightful way to take herbs. The benefit of using herbs in this way (unlike other sweet medicines), is that elixirs can be taken in small doses and reduce their impact on blood sugar. Unlike tinctures, when you make single herb extractions and then combine the extracts, with elixirs you collect a variety of herbs and mix them together. You then macerate them with equal parts of honey and brandy at the same ratio as when making tinctures.

**Dosage:** 15 drops or ½ tsp/30 drops, which you need to take every two to three hours.

# External preparations

## Herbs you can use

Most herbal constituents are absorbed readily through the external skin and the following preparations are designed to enhance this pathway into the body.

### Herbal baths

A very pleasant and simple way to take herbs is in a fragrant hot bath. There are various ways to add herbs to bath water. Dilute essential oils (one drop of essential oil per drop of base oil such as sesame) can be added. You can hang a muslin bag with fresh or dried aromatic herbs under the hot tap, or 600 ml (1 pint) as a strong herbal infusion (double or triple the standard dose described above) can be added to the water. Soak in the warm bath for 10-20 minutes.

When you use herbs in this way, the essential oils from the aromatic herbs are absorbed via the skin pores that are opened up by the warmth of the water. The oils are also carried on the steam, which is simultaneously inhaled via nose and mouth into the lungs and passing on into the bloodstream. From the nose, messages are carried from the oils via the nerve pathways to the brain.

Herbal medicines are assimilated quickly and directly, bypassing the digestive process necessary when herbs are taken by mouth. They are particularly useful for relaxing and soothing the nervous system and for easing mental and emotional strain. Lavender, basil, rose and chamomile are not only wonderfully fragrant but also relaxing, calming tension and anxiety and helping to ensure restful sleep. Chamomile is excellent for fractious children, especially when they are unwell, for not only does it possess antimicrobial properties but also helps induce sleep and is nature's best way to ward off infection and enable self healing. Rosemary baths, while also relaxing, have a stimulating edge as they enhance blood flow to the head and promote greater alertness and concentration.

### Hand and foot baths

Mustard foot baths have been used for generations to relieve all afflictions associated

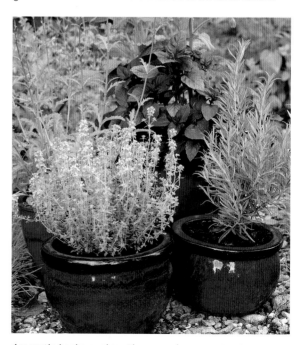

*Aromatic herbs such as thyme and rosemary can transform your bath into a therapeutic experience.*

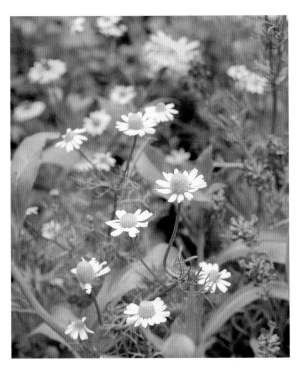

*Chamomile is an excellent herb for making creams to relieve skin problems.*

with cold and damp climates, from colds and flu to poor circulation and arthritis. The ancient tradition of hand and foot baths was made popular by the famous French herbalist, Maurice Messegue. He recommends foot baths for eight minutes in the evening and hand baths, also for eight minutes, in the morning. The hands and feet are, according to Messegue, highly sensitive areas of the skin, rich in nerve endings and despite some thickening of the skin from use, the constituents pass easily into the body.

To make hand and foot baths you can use infusions or decoctions, depending on which herbs you have selected. Alternatively you can add two to three teaspoonfuls of powdered herbs or herbal tincture to a bowl holding enough water to soak in.

## Ointments and creams

You can apply ointments and creams to treat skin problems and also less superficial problems such as inflamed joints and headaches.

Any herb, fresh or dried, can be included in an ointment following this simple recipe. Macerate as much herb as possible in 450 ml (¾ pint) of olive oil and 50 g (2 oz) of beeswax or 500 ml (17 fl oz) of pure coconut oil for a few hours over low heat in a double saucepan, after which the oil will have absorbed the constituents and you can press the mixture through a muslin bag and discard the herb. While the oil is still warm, you can pour it into ointment jars, where it will quickly solidify.

You can also make cream easily by stirring tinctures, double-strength infusions/decoctions or a few drops of essential oil into a cream base such as aqueous cream. Two to three drops of chamomile oil (matricaria chamomilla) mixed into 50 g (2 oz) of cream works well on many types of eczema.

## Compresses

Compresses can be hot or cold, depending on the symptoms. A cold compress will help reduce the swelling and pain of bruises, strains and sprains or painful joints and a hot compress will help shift congestion, reduce muscle tension and pain and improve poor circulation of blood and lymph caused by cold. They can be helpful for colds, catarrh and coughs.

You can soak a clean flannel in a hot or cold infusion or decoction, a dilute tincture or water containing a few drops of diluted essential oil, then wring it out and apply it to the affected part. This can help relieve symptoms such as

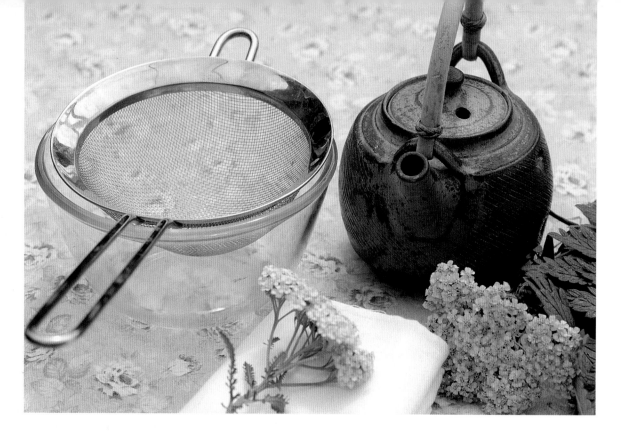

headaches, abdominal colic, backache, boils and painful joints. The treatment needs to be repeated several times to be really effective.

A 'fomentation' is basically a hot compress, generally used to treat swellings, pains, colds and flu. To prepare a fomentation, soak a cloth in the desired tea and apply it over the affected area as hot as can be tolerated. Cover the cloth with a dry flannel. Repeat as needed.

## Poultices

A poultice is very similar to a compress but involves using the herb itself. It is generally used to draw toxins from the body or from a specific area such as a boil, a splinter, an infection or swollen, painful joint, or to stimulate the circulation to the area. Some herbs, such as plantain and marshmallow, are particularly suited to this method as they have the ability to draw toxins out of the body. Other more

stimulating herbs include cayenne, garlic and rosemary. Place the herb, fresh or dried, between two pieces of gauze. If you use fresh leaves, stems or roots, they need to be chopped or bruised and softened with a little hot water before being applied. If the herbs are dry, add a little hot water to powdered or finely chopped herbs to make a paste. Use a light cotton bandage to bind the gauze poultice to the affected part and keep it warm with a hot water bottle or cover with a hot, moist towel and leave on until it cools. Repeat as often as needed, using fresh herbs.

A plaster is much like a poultice, but the herbal materials are placed between two pieces of cloth and applied to the affected area. When a herb, such as cayenne pepper or garlic, might potentially irritate the skin, this method will serve to prevent the herb from coming in direct contact with the skin.

*Opposite For compresses or formentation use a cloth soaked in herbal tea and apply it to the affected area.*

## Liniments

A rubbing oil, or liniment, consists of herb extracts in an oil or alcohol base or a mixture of both. Liniments are used in massage to relax or stimulate muscles and ligaments or to soothe away pain from inflammation or injury, joint pains, sprains and bruises.

Liniments need to be absorbed by the skin in order to reach the affected part and so they often contain stimulating herbs or essential oils such as cayenne, ginger or black pepper. For this reason they are therefore not suitable for use on delicate baby skins.

An alcohol-based liniment tends to bring out its cooling qualities, quickly evaporating and leaving the herbal properties to penetrate the skin. An oil-based liniment will stay on the skin much longer; it is also more warming.

Place your chosen herbs, coarsely chopped, in a jar. Pour in alcohol, such as vodka or brandy. Put a lid on the jar and store it in a warm, dark place for seven to ten days, shaking well at least once each day. Strain the mixture through muslin or a strainer, squeezing the herb material to get out as much of the liquid as possible. Pour it into an airtight container and label clearly.

To make an oil-based liniment, place the chopped herbs in a jar and cover with sesame, jojoba or almond oil. Cover and let stand for three days, shaking it well at least once each day. Add essential oils of your choice, two drops of essential oil per teaspoon of base oil. Follow directions as above.

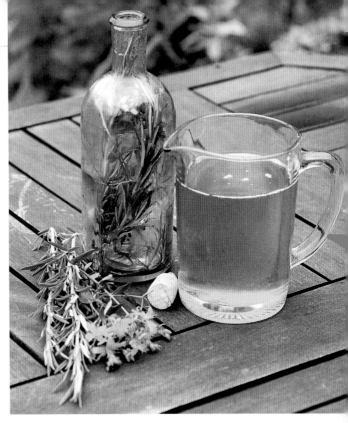

*To make an infused oil place the herbs in a glass bottle and pour over olive or sesame oil.*

## Oils

While essential oils are extracted by steam distillation from aromatic plants, you can prepare infused oils easily at home. Place finely chopped herbs in a jar, cover them with oil, such as olive or sesame, put on a tightly fitting lid and place on a sunny windowsill. Leave them to macerate for about two weeks. The oil will slowly take up the constituents of the plant.

If you macerate St John's wort in oil you will see this happening very quickly; the oil turning a deep red colour. This is a useful remedy for healing cuts and sores, and when you massage over the affected area you can relieve painful nerve conditions. After two weeks, filter the oil off and squeeze the remainder through a muslin bag. Store it in an airtight dark bottle to retain its therapeutic value for a maximum length of time.

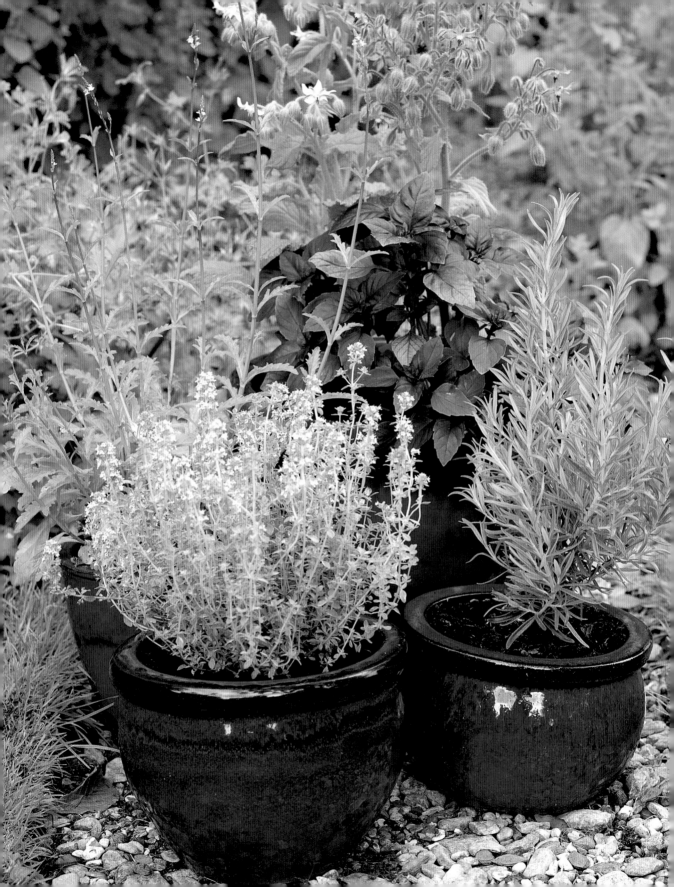

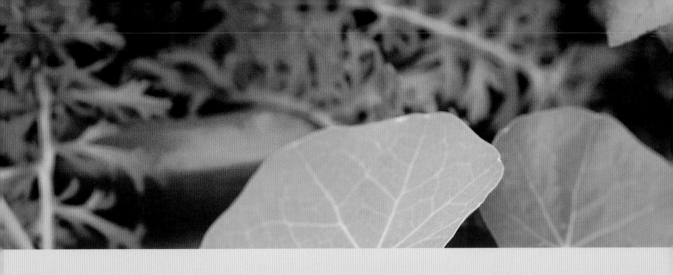

# grow your own

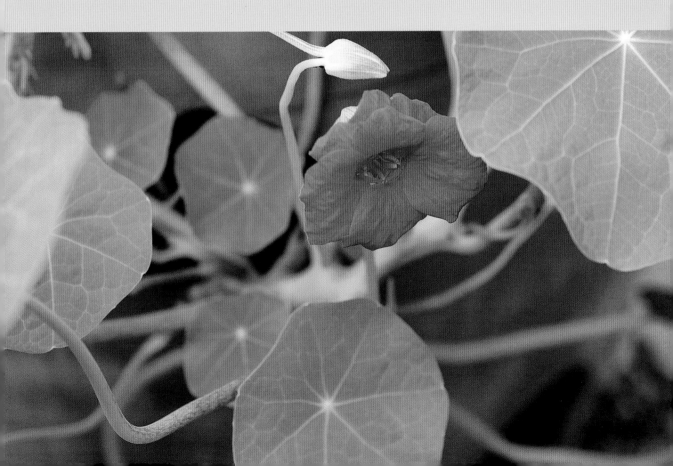

# Growing herbs
## Everything you need in pots

With their vibrant colours and delightful scents herbs are wonderfully rewarding to grow. As long as they have suitable soil and shelter from winds, most are easy to grow and you don't need specialist knowledge. You can adapt whatever space you have to growing medicinal herbs. They will thrive happily in containers on a patio, ramble up trellises, or adorn decorative pots on your windowsill. They can be planted singly, in groups or mingled with vegetables or flowers.

### Herbs in small spaces
You can easily grow herbs in containers – in window boxes, troughs, old sinks, urns or

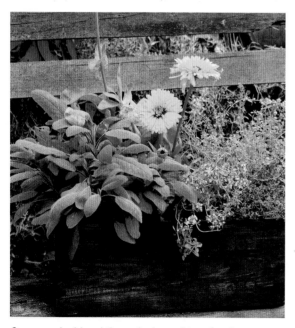

*Sage, marigold and thyme look good together in a wooden box.*

*Opposite Almost any container can be used for growing herbs, as long as it has drainage holes in the base.*

decorative pots, including strawberry pots, even teapots, but they do require a little more care than growing in open ground. Take your pick from whatever you have to hand, though container-grown herbs are prone to waterlogging from overwatering and to drying out, particularly in hot weather. They need to be fed regularly and the soil kept just moist. When choosing a planter opt for something that allows good drainage, to prevent the soil from becoming too wet. You can drill holes into the bottom of a container, such as a metal bucket. Drainage material can be gravel, sand, pebbles, crocks, or cut-up polystyrene, and must be placed at the bottom of containers before planting.

You can plant herbs in containers and hanging baskets and place them on balconies, windowsills, porches and patios, as well as indoors on windowsills – most herbs need a minimum of five to six hours' sunlight each day. Terracotta pots and herbs make very good partners. You need to make sure they are frost-proof or take them inside for the winter.

You can use either garden soil or soil-based compost in a large outdoor pot, whereas you can use a lighter compost, which you need to replenish yearly, in smaller pots. Make sure there is proper drainage in your pot before filling it with compost. When you are planting up pots

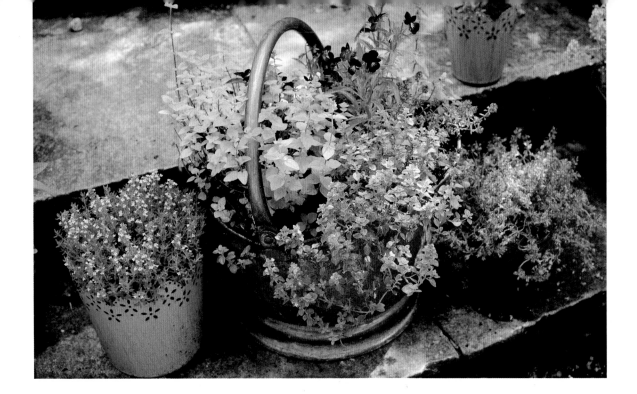

or window boxes use small herb plants or rooted cuttings and try not to cram too many plants into one pot as they will fast outgrow their space. Avoid large, vigorous-growing herbs such as lovage, angelica, comfrey, elecampane and horseradish. If you want to grow an invasive herb such as mint, tarragon, yarrow and lemon balm, the variegated varieties tend to be slower-growing. Strawberry pots have holes in the sides and are excellent for creeping, trailing herbs such as wild strawberry, creeping thyme, nasturtiums and mint.

## Planting

It is important to consider the size that a plant will grow to in your container and it is necessary to plan where you will put them. Start with the biggest one, which will usually go in the middle or middle back of your planter. Fill the container to just below the top with compost. Dig out a hole the size of the root ball of your plant then gently place the plant in position and add compost around the roots, gently firming in as you go,

enough to ensure that the plant is steady and without damaging the roots. The compost should come to just below the first shoots and for the best displays should be level or just below the top of the planter.

When growing herbs in pots you may find that they need to be replaced as they outgrow their space or become straggly. Some plants need to be lifted and protected over the winter and some faster-growing plants, such as mint, need their roots carefully monitored. It is possible to plant such plants in their existing pots to stop their roots spreading around other plant roots – cover them with compost or gravel, then they can simply be lifted out when they need replacing.

## Watering and feeding

Water the compost thoroughly after planting (or as you go if you are planting a tall, layered planter or hanging basket). It is better to water the compost directly rather than over the top of the plants, to avoid scorching. The level of the

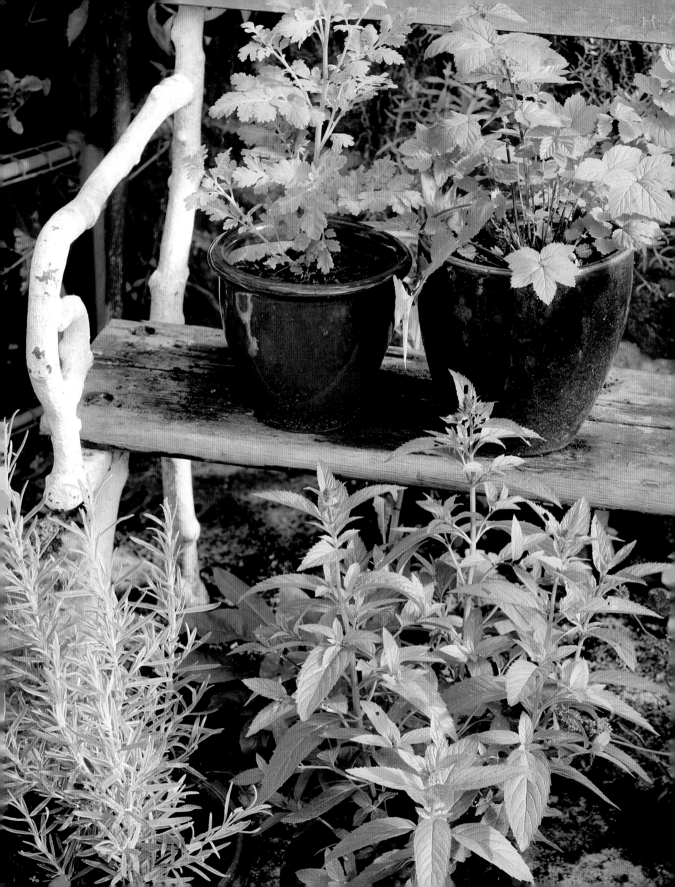

*Some fast-growing perennials, such as rosemary, peppermint and meadowsweet may require larger containers once they grow and need more space.*

compost will drop after watering, so add more to raise the level again. The container needs to be watered regularly – every day if the weather is hot and dry. To ensure a longer-lasting display, feed the plants with an organic fertilizer. Fertilizers come in different forms: liquid, powder and tablets. They are normally added to a watering can. You should feed once a week through the summer.

## Herbs on patios or paving

Many herbs look attractive planted in gaps between stones in patios, paths or paving stones, between bricks or in gravel. Low, creeping aromatic herbs are most suitable and are delightful to walk on as they release their scents when bruised or brushed against.

If you are laying a new patio be sure to leave gaps for herbs randomly, or design a more symmetrical pattern, the easiest of which is alternate paving stones and herb beds. If your patio is already in place, try removing chipped corners of stone. Squeeze a little soil in to plant a small herb. Good plants for patios are: creeping thyme, pennyroyal, marjoram, chamomile and corsican mint.

## Medicinal herbs

Medicinal herbs that can be grown in containers consist of a mixture of annuals, biennials and perennials. Annual herbs include dill, coriander, basil, German chamomile, borage and marigold and you can grow these easily from seed. Biennials take two summers to flower, usually producing an attractive rosette of leaves in the

first year. They include caraway, mullein, and evening primrose. Herbaceous perennials continue from one year to the next, dying down in autumn and reappearing the next spring. They can mostly be grown from seed, but may be easier to grow from root division, planting cuttings or offsets.

Herbs grown in pots can be planted at most times of the year, except when the earth is frozen or snow-covered, and provided they are healthy they will easily establish themselves. Always ensure you choose strong, healthy-looking plants, free from disease or insects and avoid straggly plants and those with roots escaping from the bottom of the pot. Also make sure that the plants are clearly labelled. Some fast-growing perennials may have to be moved once they grow and need more space. Try to avoid planting new pot herbs in dry, hot weather and be sure to keep the plants watered well until they are well established.

## Planning your herb planting

Many medicinal herbs originate in warm climates and so to grow happily in temperate climes they prefer sheltered positions. If your growing area is warm and sheltered there is no need to enclose it and herbs can be planted in the open. Before planting your containers it is a good idea to plan your planting design. Take into account the aspect of the area, related to sun or shade. Most herbs like to grow in warm, sheltered and sunny positions, while some prefer light shade.

Lavender, basil, juniper, bay, rosemary, coriander, sage, hyssop, thyme and marjoram prefer full sun, while angelica, lovage, wild strawberry, borage, mint, chives, parsley, fennel, pennyroyal, lemon balm, ground ivy prefer dappled shade. Comfrey, valerian, lungwort, violet, tansy and mint prefer full shade. If your area is exposed to wind and weather fencing could make all the difference.

Choose the herbs that suit you best and make a list of them. Check their height and the time of year when they will look decorative to decide on their positions. This will ensure that they look good for as long as possible through the changing seasons. Low-growing plants such as marjoram, thyme, marigolds (calendula), basil and wood betony will be best planted near the front of your containers, and taller ones, such as lavender, rosemary, rose, borage and fennel should go at the back. Herbs such as sage, thyme, rosemary, and marjoram establish themselves surprisingly quickly.

### Sowing seeds

You can buy herb seeds from suppliers or you can save your own from the previous year. Sow early plants as seed in pots or trays in a propagator in early spring. Using fresh seedling compost sow the seeds evenly by sprinkling them over the firmed soil or in shallow drills. Cover the seeds lightly with a thin layer of compost or fine sand and water. Label and cover with a piece of glass or sheet of newspaper until germination.

When the seedlings are large enough to handle, thin them or transplant them to pots. Once they have become sturdy plant them outdoors in early summer. Alternatively, sow seeds directly into warmer soil in pots outside in late spring or early summer once all sign of frost has gone. Cover the seeds with soil, the depth of which can be measured by multiplying the diameter of the seeds two to three times.

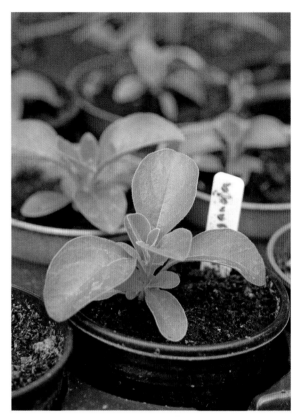

*Once the seedlings are sturdy they can be planted outdoors in their pots.*

Growing herbs from seed is highly rewarding, particularly if you have collected them yourself. In addition, you may find that your own seeds germinate more successfully than bought ones. You can sow them in trays and leave them in a cold frame covered with a piece of polythene until they germinate, which may not happen until the following spring.

Many variegated herbs and decorative, coloured herbs, such as purple and golden sages, will not come true when you grow them from seed and so they need to be propagated by cuttings or root division. Many herbs self-seed freely if their seed heads are left alone. These include evening primrose, lady´s mantle, chamomile, coriander, marigold and motherwort. Seeds will germinate when conditions are right and will develop into strong, healthy plants. If they grow in places where you don´t want them you can easily move them when they are ready.

### Root division

Herbs that form good clumps are excellent for root division and examples such as chives, bergamot, catmint, valerian, tarragon and yarrow need to be divided every three or four years into smaller clumps for the best results. It is best to carry out all root division in autumn or early spring. First cut back the top growth and dig up the entire plant. Carefully divide the clump into several pieces, each retaining a good system of roots, and replant.

### Taking cuttings

Taking cuttings from established plants is an easy way to propagate herbs. Softwood, semi-ripe and hardwood cuttings can be taken, depending on the plant. Soft tip cuttings are generally successful with most herbaceous perennials, while semi-ripe and hardwood cuttings are suitable for shrubs such as sage and rosemary.

When you are taking cuttings, gently tear a small side-shoot off a stem so that it has a heel on it, or cut the shoot´s stem just below a leaf joint. Remove the lower leaves and insert them into holes around the edge of a pot of cutting compost, or a mixture of peat and sand.

Firm the soil around the cuttings and water in well. Use your hand to do this. Once you see signs of new growth at the tip, lift each cutting gently and plant up in individual pots.

### Softwood cuttings

It is best to take softwood cutting in spring and early summer from healthy looking plants. Once inserted around the edge of your pot or tray, spray the cuttings with water and cover with polythene to retain moisture. Roots develop quickly on softwood cuttings, generally within three to six weeks, but less in warm conditions. Root development stimulates leaf growth so you will know roots are formed when you see new leaves shooting at the growing tip. Once the root system is established lift the cutting and pot it up individually or plant in a nursery bed. Generally, it is best to keep them in pots in a sheltered area, or indoors in cold areas during the first winter and plant them outside the following spring.

### Semi-ripe cuttings

These are taken in summer when stems are harder as they ripen at the base but are still flexible. Side shoots are taken off the new growth, torn away from the main stem, leaving a little heel of older wood. Once inserted in pots or trays and watered in, they are also best covered with polythene to retain moisture, but it is not vital as they are more resilient than soft wood cuttings. Keep in pots in a cold frame or a sheltered area out of direct sunlight until growth starts the following spring.

### Hardwood cuttings

These are taken from shrubby herbs such as bay, southernwood, rosemary, and sage in autumn once the plant is dormant. Take a side shoot of the current year´s growth up to 30 cm (12 in), remove lower leaves and insert half their length in compost in light soil in the garden in a sheltered position. Firm the soil around the cutting and water well. Leave for around a year until a good root system is developed.

### Root cuttings or offsets

This is the ideal method of propagation for herbs that have running roots or that send up side shoots, such as yarrow, chamomile, mint, pennyroyal, and valerian. Cut the spreading roots or runners from the parent plant at the end of summer or early autumn. Cut the root into small pieces about 5 cm (2 in) long and put them on compost with a little sand in a seed tray. Cover with plastic and leave in a cold frame, greenhouse, tunnel or sheltered spot. Once new shoots appear remove the plastic and plant out.

### Layering and mounding

You can propagate low-growing and shrubby herbs such as sage, thyme, lavender, periwinkle by layering. Take a low-growing branch and fix it in contact with the soil. Once a root has developed separate the new plant, dig it up and replant. Spreading herbs such as chamomile, thyme, pennyroyal can be partially covered with soil in their centre; a process called 'mounding', so bringing different parts of the plant into contact with the soil. Once rooted, lots of new plants can be separated off.

### Harvesting herbs

When harvesting herbs it is important to establish which part of the plant you need – the leaves, flowers, root, rhizome or seeds and when is the best time to harvest that part. Generally, it is best to harvest the aromatic leaves of herbs, such as basil, thyme, sage, mint, lemon balm when the flowers are about to open, as essential oil content is highest then. Choose a dry day, once the dew has dried. During the growing season it is best to gather leaves and flowers and use them fresh, ideally straight from their pots. It is best to pick flowers and flowering tops such as St John's wort, agrimony, golden rod, yarrow,

skullcap and hyssop, as they are about to bloom. Put them in a flat basket to avoid bruising. Harvest some extras for drying or freezing to last through the winter. Particularly valuable are herbs that could be useful for treating winter colds and coughs, such as hyssop, thyme, oregano, ground ivy and mullein, and fevers, such as chamomile, yarrow and elderflowers. You can pick herbs such as coriander leaves, mint, sage, rosemary, parsley, chives, basil and fennel, which you may want to use freshly in the kitchen throughout the growing season.

Seeds such as dill, coriander, fennel and caraway, need to be caught when ripe, before they drop. Cut off the whole flower head, tie it up in a muslin or paper bag and hang it upside down in a well-ventilated, dry room. As the flower head dries the seeds will drop into the bag. Store the seeds in envelopes, foil or small boxes with well-fitting lids, and label clearly with the name and collection date.

It is best to harvest roots and rhizomes, such as valerian, dandelion, elecampane, burdock, when the aerial parts have died down in autumn or before growing recommences in spring, as they are richest in stored food then. When harvesting, choose healthy-looking plants. Make sure they are growing away from areas that have been sprayed or polluted. Pick only what you need at the time, as they will easily spoil and be wasted. Harvest just a few leaves and flowers from each plant so as not to threaten its health or survival.

### Drying herbs

The object of drying is to reduce or eliminate the moisture in the herb quickly, before it starts to die, so that it can be stored for a few months without deteriorating. When harvesting flowers

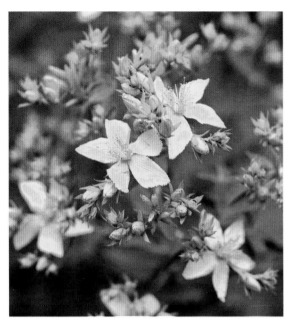

*St John's wort is best picked just as the flowers are about to burst into bloom.*

and leaves for storage make sure they are dry and pick them before the heat of the day reaches its peak. Use your fingers to pick, unless stalks, such as agrimony or yarrow, are very tough. Pick gently, taking care not to bruise the plant. When lifting roots, dig them up, trying not to puncture the outer skin. Wash the soil off and cut off any leaves left and chop up into sections or slices to speed drying and lay them out to dry.

### Best locations
Providing that herbs are dried properly, those dried at home are often of a much higher quality than shop-bought herbs in terms of colour, flavour and healing properties. Drying needs to occur quickly and evenly. Shade, air and constant warmth are essential. The best places for drying are a shaded, well-ventilated room, airing cupboard or shed, free from moisture or condensation. Avoid the kitchen, bathroom, utility room, damp sheds or garages if they are damp, as the herbs will not dry properly and will deteriorate. A steady temperature of about 32°C (90°F) is ideal. If the atmosphere is too cold (below 22°C/72°F) the plants will reabsorb moisture and take too long to dry.

### Hanging and storing
You can loosely tie aerial parts of herbs in small bunches by their stems and hang them indoors. In warm, dry climates bunches can be hung outside in the shade or from a high ceiling in a warm room with windows open, though the temperature varies through 24 hours. More reliable results may be obtained by spreading herbs over a tray, wire netting, box lid, fruit tray, drying frame, sheets of paper or muslin. Spread out the herbs and turn them once or twice the first day, and then daily. Large-leaved herbs will dry more quickly if the leaves are stripped from the stems. Always dry herbs separately.

Before storing herbs check that they are dry by seeing if they are brittle and rustle, crumble or snap easily. If herbs are stored before they are dry they will reabsorb moisture and deteriorate. It takes three to seven days for most herbs to dry. Herbs are best stored in clearly labelled, air-tight dark containers, wooden or cardboard boxes, paper bags or jars – glass jars are ideal kept in a dark cupboard, as light will cause deterioration. Never store in plastic as it encourages condensation. Remove stalks and twigs from aerial parts and break roots, rhizomes and barks into small pieces. Store seeds in packets in the fridge or air-tight jars. Some herbs, particularly those with soft leaves, such as marjoram, borage, comfrey and coriander are ideal for freezing. Pick the leaves or flowers, wash them and put them in small plastic bags in the freezer.

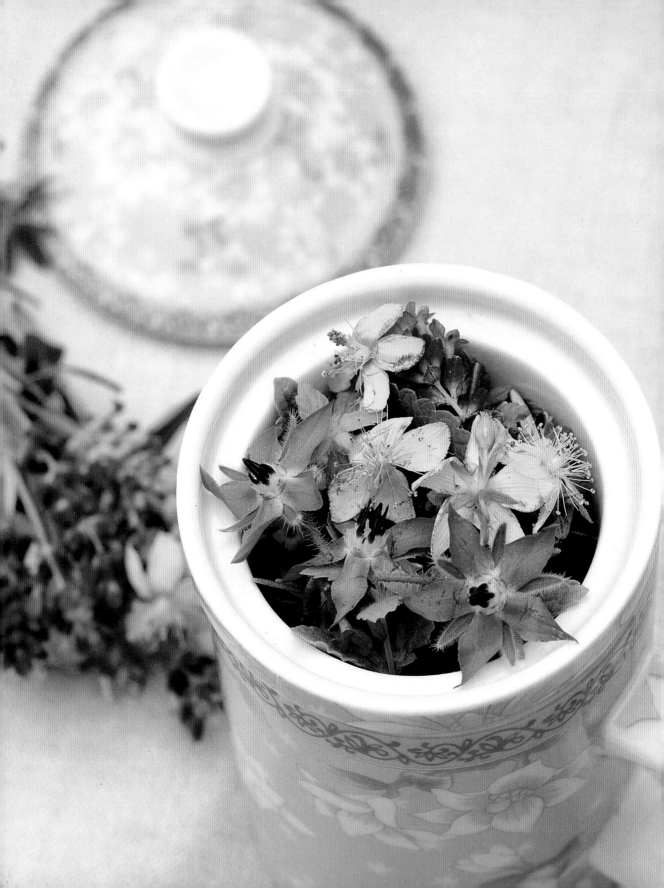

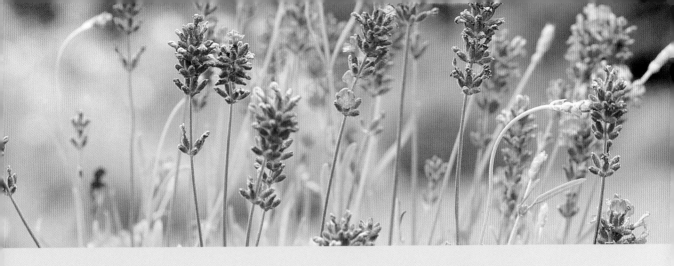

# the remedies

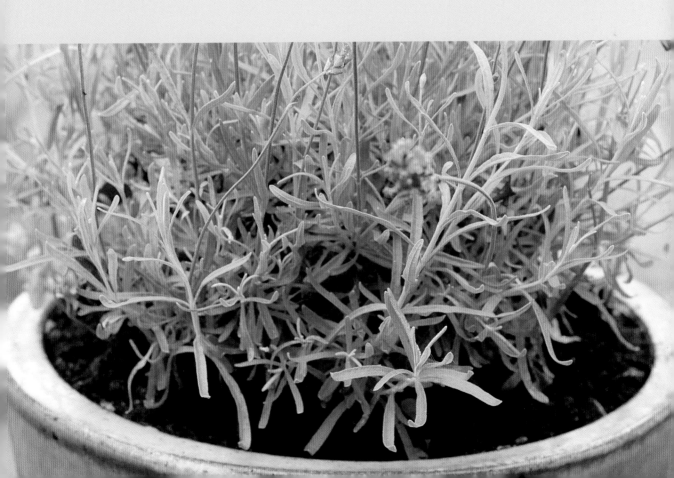

# Steaming foot bath

## For colds and flu

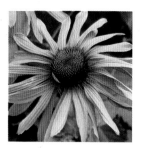

Soaking your feet in a hot herbal bath is a favourite remedy for the first signs of infection, relieving aches and pains, reducing fevers and clearing catarrh. This aromatic combination will help fight infection, reduce swelling of mucous membranes, loosen and clear catarrh.

## Ingredients

- 3 teaspoons each fresh or 2 teaspoons dried leaves peppermint, yarrow, garlic, echinacea, nasturtium
- 1¼ litres (2½ pints) boiling water

Makes 1¼ litres (2½ pints) infusion

## How to make

**1** Make a strong infusion by pouring boiling water over the herb mixture.
**2** Cover and let the mixture stand for at least 30 minutes and then strain.

## How to use

Pour into a bowl and when the infusion is cool enough, soak your feet for 10–15 minutes 3 times a day. You can also drink it as a tisane every hour or two for swift relief.

## GROWING

Place drainage material in the base of a strawberry pot. Fill with compost to the first level of holes in the sides and plant two peppermints and two nasturtiums through the holes. Add more compost up to the next holes and plant two more peppermints and two nasturtiums, alternating them to produce a cascade of colour for an effective visual display. Water at each level of planting. Plant the yarrow, garlic and echinacea in the top. Water well and feed weekly.

### Plants you will need

- 4 *Mentha piperita* (peppermint)
- 4 *Tropaeolum majus* (nasturtium)
- 1 *Achillea millefolium* (yarrow)
- 3 *Allium sativum* (garlic)
- 1 *Echinacea angustifolia* (purple coneflower)

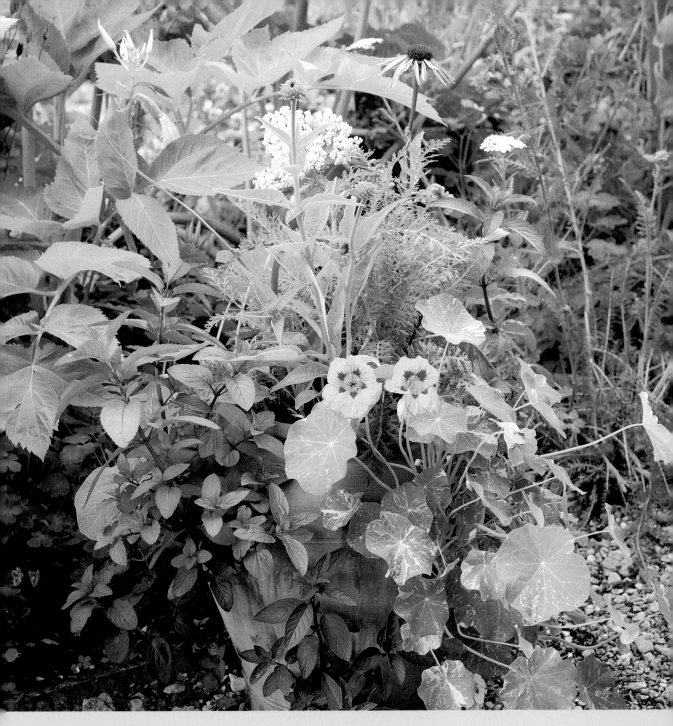

## You could also try...

Using a mustard foot bath similarly ♦ Drinking hot ginger tea or hot lemon with honey 3–4 times daily ♦ Taking supplements of 500 mg vitamin C every 2 hours and 15 mg of zinc daily ♦ Drinking teas of other immune-enhancing and decongestant herbs including dill, lemon balm, chamomile, lavender, thyme, rosemary, elderberries and flowers, cinnamon, cardamom, turmeric and coriander through the day.

# Breathe-easy inhalation

## For catarrh

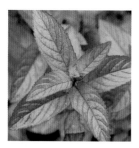

Inhaling the aromatic steam from a hot peppermint, thyme and nasturtium tea is a really effective way to clear the airways. Peppermint is a well-known decongestant, while thyme and nasturtium are warming and stimulating, helping to fight off infection and clear catarrh.

## Ingredients

- 3 teaspoons each fresh or 2 teaspoons dried of thyme, peppermint and nasturtium
- 1¼ litres (2½ pints) boiling water

Makes 1¼ litres (2½ pints) tea

## How to make

**1** Place the herbs in a teapot.
**2** Pour over the boiling water and leave to stand for 15 minutes.
**3** Strain through a fine mesh strainer and pour into a bowl.

## How to use

Place the bowl on a firm surface, cover your head with a towel and inhale the wonderful aromas for about 10 minutes or until you feel your nose and chest clearing. Repeat 2 or 3 times a day.

**Did you know?**
Peppermint contains menthol oils and is a penetrating decongestant.

## GROWING

Line the hanging basket with moss or a similar permeable membrane to allow for drainage. Cover the lining with enough compost to reach the top of the basket. Place the peppermint in the centre, surround it with four nasturtiums alternated with the thyme. Water regularly and feed weekly.

**Plants you will need**

- 1 *Mentha piperita* (peppermint)
- 4 *Tropaeolum majus* (nasturtium)
- 3 *Thymus vulgaris* (thyme)

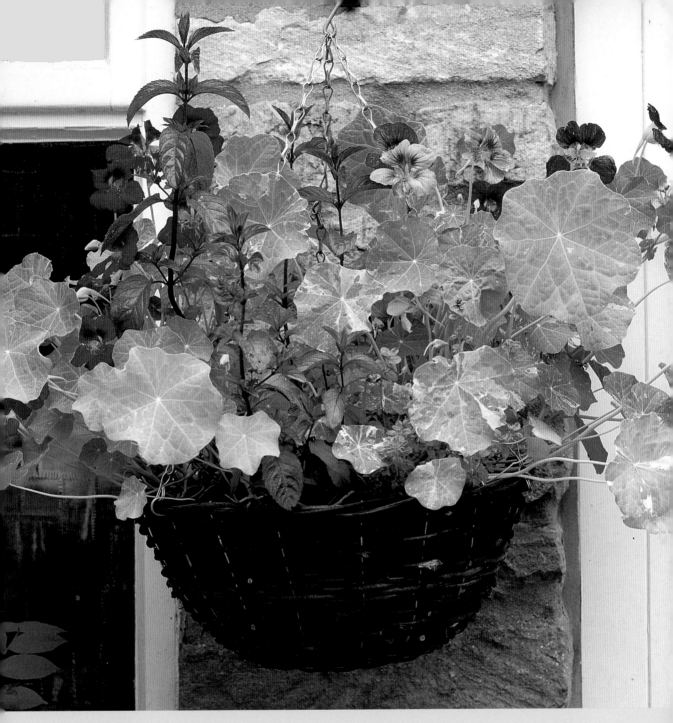

## You could also try...

Inhaling oils of lavender, rosemary, ginger, cinnamon or chamomile, adding them to baths or massage oils for around the nose and sinuses ♦ Washing the sinuses by sniffing salt water ♦ Omitting wheat, dairy and sugar from the diet ♦ Drinking teas of the herbs above or of echinacea, thyme, ginger, cinnamom, yarrow, chamomile, agrimony or meadowsweet 3–6 times daily.

# Soothing herbal honey
## For coughs

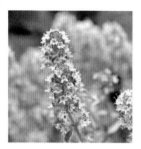

Honey has antibacterial, expectorant and healing properties, so herbal honeys are good for coughs and chest infections and an excellent medium for antimicrobial and expectorant herbs thyme, oregano, and holy basil. All these herbs taste delicious and are good decongestants.

## Ingredients

- 500 g (1 lb) jar organic runny honey
- 4 teaspoons each fresh or 2 teaspoons dried purple basil, thyme, marjoram

**Makes enough to fill a 500 g (1 lb) jar**

## How to make

**1** Fill the jar with the herbs. You can use a reusable teabag or tie the herbs into a piece of muslin if you like.

**2** Cover them with honey and close with an airtight lid, label clearly and leave to macerate for at least 4 weeks.

**3** Remove the herbs, label clearly with name and date and store in a cool, dark place, preferably the fridge.

## How to use

Take 1 teaspoon daily in a cup of hot water or ginger tea as a preventative and 3–6 times daily for acute infections. Children love it!

## GROWING

Place a layer of moss/padding in the bottom of each metal basket and then fill with multipurpose compost. Plant the thyme in the bottom, the oregano in the next layer and basil at the top. Water regularly, but do not overwater as these Mediterranean plants prefer slightly dry soil and feed weekly.

### Plants you will need

- 3 *Thymus vulgaris* (thyme)
- 2 *Origanum majorana* (marjoram)
- 5 *Ocimum basilicum* 'Purpurascens' (purple basil)

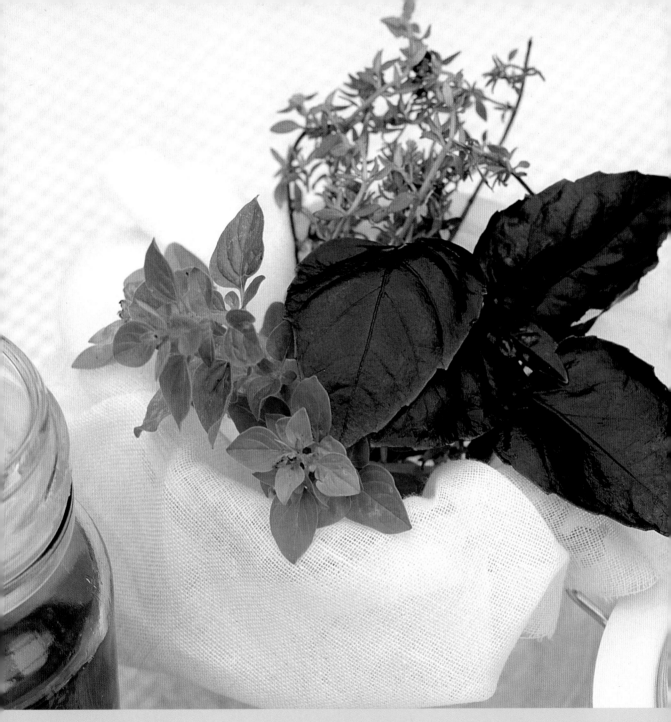

## You could also try...

Drinking a tisane using the same herbs 3–6 times daily ♦ Drinking other soothing, antimicrobial and expectorant teas including mullein, plantain, licorice, coltsfoot, elecampane, ground ivy, ginger or rose petals ♦ Taking supplements of vitamin C and eating garlic, elderberries and bilberries to clear phlegm and combat infection ♦ Using oils of rosemary, rose, thyme, ginger, or cinnamon for herbal baths.

# Fiery gargle
## For sore throats

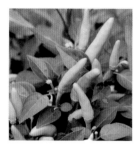

Red sage and cayenne pepper make a colourful combination with their hues of purple and red. Gargling with sage is a great way to ease a sore throat and stop infection. Cayenne is also an excellent antiseptic and analgesic, helping to relieve soreness and pain.

## Ingredients

- 4 teaspoons fresh or 2 teaspoons dried sage leaves
- small slice cayenne pepper or pinch dried chilli powder
- pinch sea salt
- 200 ml (7 fl oz) boiling water
- 2 tablespoons each honey and apple cider vinegar

Makes 200 ml (7 fl oz) gargle

## How to make

**1** Place the sage and cayenne in a jug then pour over the boiling water.
**2** Cover and leave to infuse for 10–15 minutes and then add a pinch of salt, which helps fight off infection.
**3** Add the cider vinegar and honey and stir well.

## How to use

Gargle with half a cupful 3–6 times a day or use the mixture in a throat spray and the pain will soon ease.

### Did you know?
Apple cider vinegar makes a great medium for this gargle because it is both antiviral and antibacterial.

## GROWING

Fill the bottom of a medium-sized round pot with drainage material and top up with a multipurpose compost. Plant the red sage in early summer in the back, and the cayenne pepper in front, once all danger of frost has passed. Water regularly and feed weekly.

### Plants you will need

- 1 *Salvia officinalis* (red sage)
- 1 *Capsicum frutescens* (cayenne pepper)

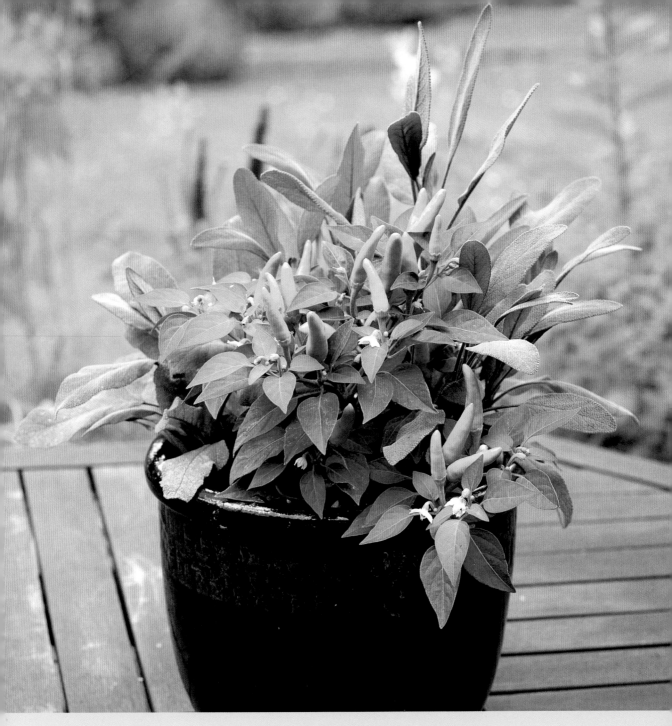

## You could also try...

Applying a hot compress made from a strong infusion of equal parts of red sage leaves, calendula petals and plantain leaves frequently to the throat

♦ Drinking teas of antimicrobial herbs such as echinacea, turmeric, cat's claw, pau d'arco, licorice, calendula, burdock, or red clover every 2 hours

♦ Taking supplements of garlic, cod liver oil, vitamin C and zinc.

# Cooling tisane

## For fevers

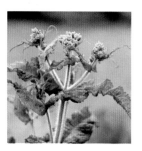

This delicious combination can be prepared as an infusion and drunk as a tea, used as a foot bath and as a tepid wash to cool the body. The herbs used enhance immunity, fight off infection, bring down fevers and help you sleep. They are also relaxing, antimicrobial and decongestant.

## Ingredients

- 2 teaspoons each fresh or 1 teaspoon dried chamomile, purple basil, boneset, yarrow, peppermint and lemon balm
- 1¼ litres (2½ pints) water

Makes 1¼ litres (2½ pints) tisane

## How to make

**1** Place the herbs in a teapot. Pour over boiling water.
**2** Cover and leave to infuse for 10–15 minutes.

## How to use

Drink a cupful every hour or two. You can also pour the tea into a bowl and, when it is cool enough, soak your feet in it for 10 minutes every 2–3 hours.

**Did you know?**
Boneset enhances immunity and is famous as a flu remedy, promoting sweating and clearing heat and toxins.

## GROWING

Cover the bottom of three pots of matching colour with drainage material and top up with a multipurpose compost. Plant the boneset in the middle of the largest pot, the chamomile around it and the purple basil in front. Plant the lemon balm and peppermint in the second pot and the yarrow in the third. Water regularly and feed weekly.

**Plants you will need**

- 1 *Eupatorium perfoliatum* (boneset)
- 4 *Matricaria recutita* (German chamomile) or *Anthemis nobilis/Chamaemelum nobile* (Roman chamomile)
- 1 *Ocimum basilicum* 'Purpurascens' (purple basil)
- 1 *Melissa officinalis* (lemon balm)
- 3 *Mentha piperita* (peppermint)
- 1 *Achillea millefolium* (yarrow)

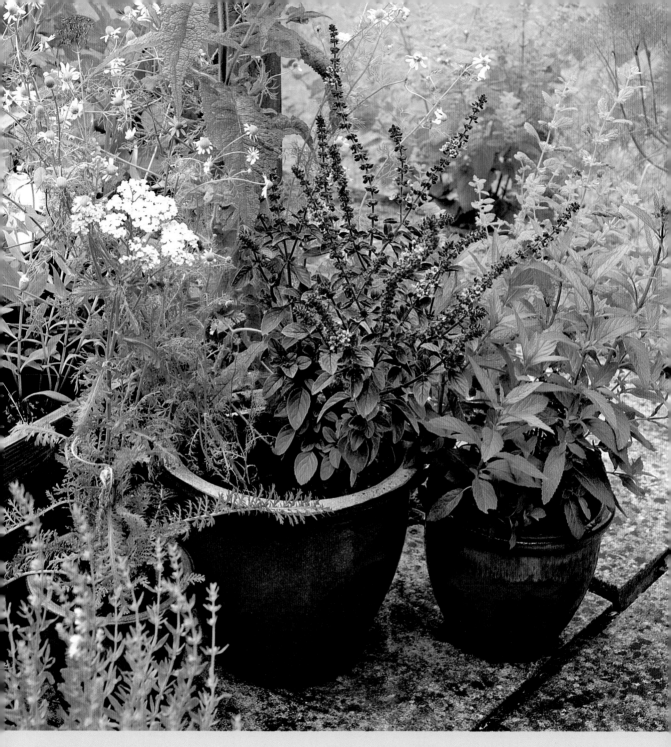

## You could also try...

Fasting to boost the immune system ♦ Drinking plenty of fluids to help elimination of toxins ♦ Drinking teas of limeflower, meadowsweet, vervain, rose, elderflower, lavender or ginger 3–6 times daily ♦ Taking ½ teaspoon echinacea every 2 hours to help fight off infection.

# Antihistamine mix

## For hay fever

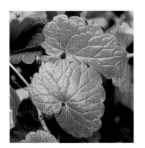

This multicoloured assortment makes a pleasant remedy when hay fever spoils your summer. Echinacea, chamomile and lemon balm soothe the allergic response that sparks off symptoms, while agrimony and ground ivy calm inflammation, drying up secretions.

## Ingredients

• 400 ml (14 fl oz) plant glycerol
• 100 ml (3½ fl oz) alcohol (vodka or brandy)
• 250 g (9 oz) each fresh or 100 g (3½ oz) dried agrimony, chamomile, echinacea, lemon balm and ground ivy

Makes enough to fill a 500 ml (17 fl oz) jar

## How to make

**1** First mix the glycerol and alcohol together.
**2** Place the herbs in a wide-necked jar and pour the mixture over the herbs.
**3** Leave to macerate for at least 2–3 weeks, stirring daily and then strain through a fine mesh sieve or muslin or press using a wine press, making sure that you squeeze as much liquid from the herbs as possible.
**4** Pour into dark, sterilized bottles, label carefully and store in a cool, dark place.

## How to use

Take a teaspoon 3–6 times daily in a little water, depending on the severity of the symptoms.

## GROWING

Cover the bottom of a window box with drainage material and top up with a multipurpose compost. Plant the ground ivy at one end of the planter and the chamomile at the other. Place the lemon balm in the centre and the echinacea and agrimony at either side. Water regularly and feed weekly.

### Plants you will need

• 1 *Glechoma/Nepeta hederacea* (ground ivy)
• 3 *Matricaria recutita* (German chamomile) or *Anthemis nobilis/Chamaemelum nobile* (Roman chamomile)
• 1 *Melissa officinalis* (lemon balm)
• 1 *Echinacea angustifolia* (purple coneflower)
• 1 *Agrimonia eupatoria* (agrimony)

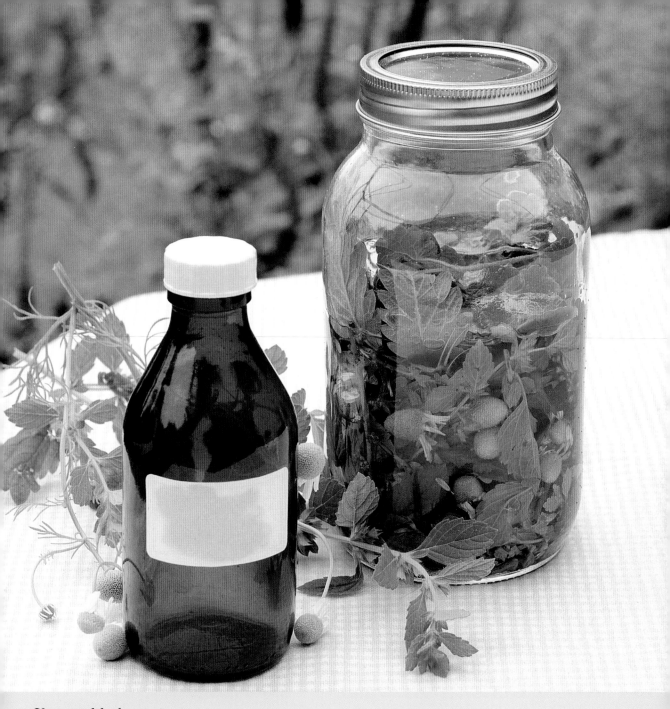

## You could also try...

Taking immune enhancing herbs as preventatives 2–4 months before the hay fever season, such as ashwagandha, Siberian ginseng or echinacea ✦ Taking 1–2 tablespoons of local honey in honeycombs with each meal for 2–4 months before the hayfever season ✦ Cutting out wheat and dairy ✦ Using these herbs as teas for inhalations ✦ Drinking teas of elderflower, plantain and eyebright ✦ Taking supplements of evening primrose oil, vitamin C and magnesium ✦ Wearing sunglasses to reduce eye irritation.

# Aromatic honey

## For asthma

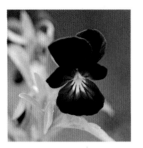

This honey is excellent for coughs and asthma. Thyme and marjoram relax bronchial muscles, clear mucus, dispel infection and open the airways. Basil is a calming herb, clearing congestion and relaxing chest muscles. Wild pansy is good for bronchitis, coughs, asthma and catarrh.

## Ingredients

♦ 1–2 cups each fresh or ½–1 cup dried purple basil leaves, thyme flowers and leaves, marjoram leaves, wild pansy flowers and leaves
♦ 400 ml (14 fl oz) honey, either thyme or Manuka honey

**Makes enough to fill a 400 ml (14 fl oz) jar**

## How to make

**1** Add the herbs directly to the honey, or use a reusable teabag or muslin bag to contain the herbs.
**2** Heat the mixture on the stove in a double boiler for 4–5 hours and then strain it. Remove the teabag and pour into a jar.
**3** Store in a cool, dark place, preferably the fridge.

## How to use

Take 1–2 teaspoons herbal honey in a little hot water or off the spoon 3 times a day and every 2 hours in acute phases. Herbs may need to be taken over several months if the asthma is chronic.

## GROWING

Cover the bottom of a large pot with drainage material and top up with multipurpose compost. Place the plants in an attractive grouping. Deadhead the wild pansy so that it keeps flowering. Water carefully as thyme and marjoram are Mediterranean plants and prefer dry soil. Feed weekly.

**Plants you will need**

♦ 1 *Viola tricolor* (wild pansy)
♦ 2 *Thymus vulgaris* (thyme)
♦ 1 *Origanum majorana* (marjoram)

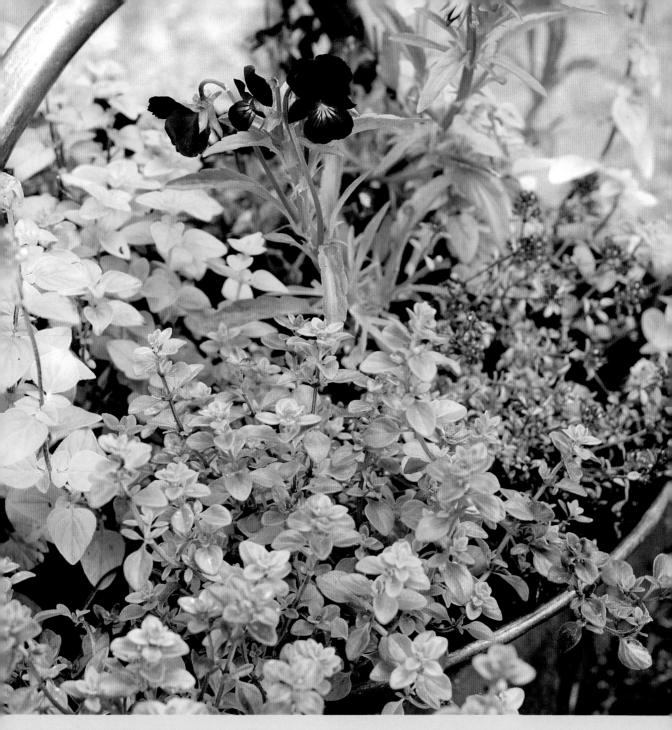

## You could also try...

Drinking teas of expectorant herbs such as elecampane, coltsfoot, ginger, licorice and mullein 3 times daily ♦ Taking ashwagandha, licorice, chamomile, nettles, holy basil, shiitake or reishi mushrooms to enhance immunity and reduce the allergic response ♦ Making lozenges with the herbs by rolling powdered herbs in honey to make a paste, which can be rolled into balls.

# Fragrant salve

## For eczema

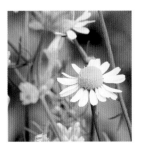

This smooth cream, made from chamomile, marigold (calendula) and lavender, can soothe and heal. Chamomile is anti-inflammatory, while marigold cools inflammation, speeding healing and helping to prevent infection. Delicate lavender can heal without scarring and is antiseptic.

## Ingredients

- 300 ml (10 fl oz) coconut oil, warmed
- Fresh or dry marigold petals, chamomile flowers and lavender flowers (as much as will fit into the oil and remain submerged)

Makes 300 ml (10 fl oz) salve

## How to make

**1** Pour the warmed coconut oil into a double saucepan.
**2** Chop the herbs roughly and submerge them in the oil.
**3** Leave to macerate for a few hours over low heat, after which the oil will have absorbed the constituents, and then press the mixture through a muslin bag. Discard the herbs.

**4** While the oil is still warm, pour it into sterilized ointment jars, where it will quickly solidify. Label them clearly and store in a cool place.

## How to use

Apply the cream night and morning, after gently washing the area with rose water.

## GROWING

Cover the bottom of a large circular pot with drainage material, then top up with a multipurpose compost. In early summer plant the lavender in the centre and the marigold (calendula) and chamomile plants alternately round it, leaving plenty of space for growth. Deadhead the marigolds so that they flower repeatedly. Water regularly and feed weekly.

### Plants you will need

- 1 *Lavandula officinalis* (lavender)
- 4 *Calendula officinalis* (marigold)
- 4 *Matricaria recutita* (German chamomile) or *Anthemis nobilis/Chamaemelum nobile* (Roman chamomile)

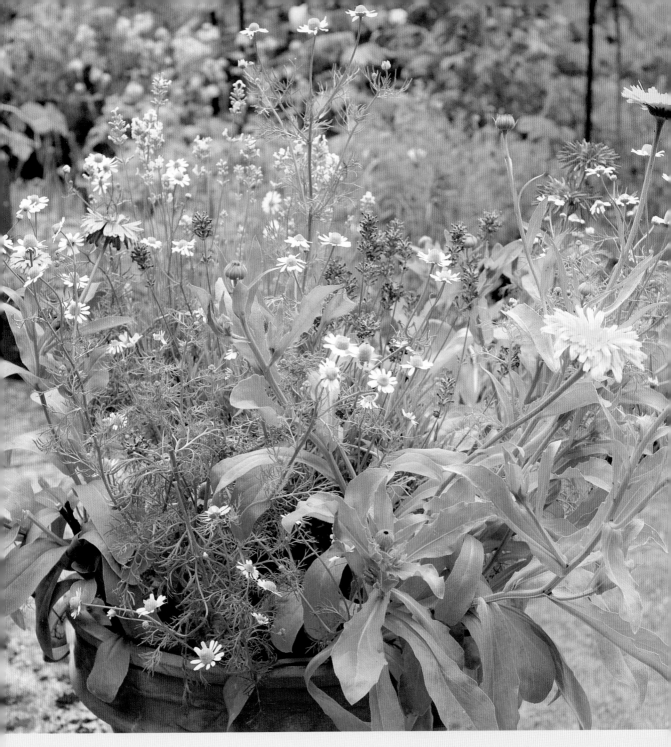

## You could also try...

Drinking teas made from the same herbs 3–4 times a day ♦ Drinking teas of cleavers, burdock, gotu kola, dandelion root or red clover 3–4 times daily ♦ Avoiding dairy produce, wheat, junk foods and sugar ♦ Taking supplements of evening primrose oil, vitamin-B complex and zinc.

# Cleansing skin wash

## For acne

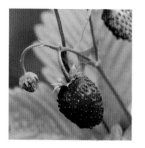

The bright-blue flowers of borage and the sweet faces of wild pansies lend this recipe eye appeal. Both are cleansing, while young dandelion leaves help clear the skin. Nasturtium leaves are antiseptic and rich in sulphur, excellent for infection and inflammation.

## Ingredients

♦ 2 teaspoons each fresh or 1 teaspoon dried wild pansy, nasturtium and borage leaves and flowers, dandelion and strawberry leaves, lavender flowers
♦ 1¼ litres (2½ pints) boiling water

**Makes 1¼ litres (2½ pints) infusion**

## How to make

Place the herbs in a teapot. Pour over the boiling water and leave to infuse until cool before straining.

## How to use

Use as an antiseptic cleanser to bathe the face night and morning.

### Did you know?

Lavender combats infection and speeds healing of scars, while strawberry leaves are anti-inflammatory and tone the skin, slowing the production of oil.

## GROWING

Cover the bottom of three matching pots with drainage material then top up with a multipurpose compost. Plant the borage in the centre of the large pot and surround it with four nasturtiums. Place the lavender in the middle of the medium-sized pot with four wild pansies around it. Place the wild strawberry and dandelions in the last pot. Deadhead the nasturtiums and wild pansies so that they keep flowering. Water regularly and feed weekly.

### Plants you will need

♦ 1 *Borago officinalis* (borage)
♦ 4 *Tropaeolum majus* (nasturtium)
♦ 1 *Lavandula officinalis* (lavender)
♦ 4 *Viola tricolor* (wild pansy)
♦ 1 *Fragaria vesca* (wild strawberry)
♦ 3 *Taraxacum officinale* (dandelion)

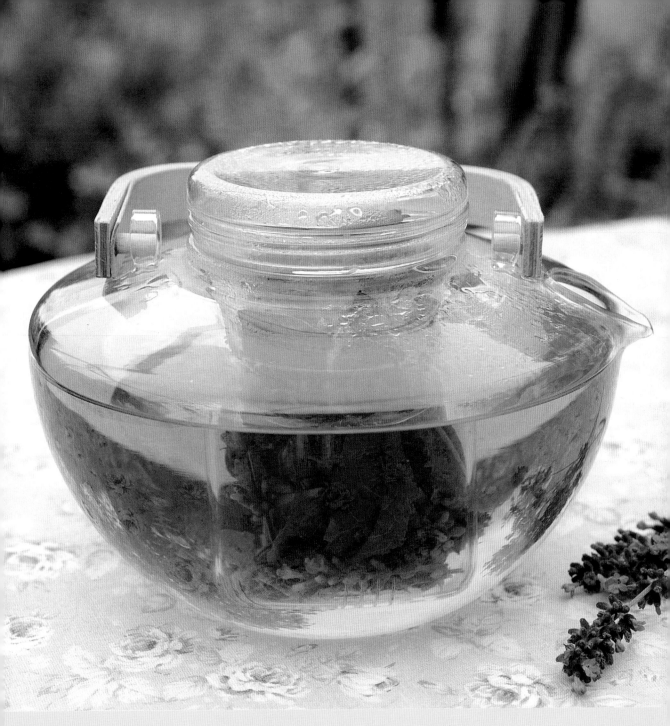

## You could also try...

Filling a wide-necked flask with equal parts of the herbs, covering with spring water and leaving to infuse overnight. Drink at least 3–4 cups of the water daily ♦ Drinking teas of milk thistle, dandelion root, burdock, rose, gotu kola, nettle or red clover 4–5 times a day ♦ Eating plenty of fresh fruit and vegetables ♦ Taking supplements of cod liver oil, vitamin-B complex and zinc.

# Fresh celandine juice
## For warts and corns

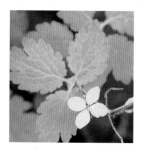

Greater celandine is an old folk remedy for warts and it really works. This member of the poppy family has cheerful flowers, which bloom through the summer. The bright-orange latex exuding from the leaf stems and flowers has an amazing ability to make warts disappear.

## Ingredients

* leaves, stem and flowers of greater celandine

## How to make

Slice the stem of the fresh plant and allow the bright-orange juice to seep out.

**Did you know?**
The latex contains proteolytic enzymes, which explains its ability to wear down warts and moles.

## How to use

Apply the juice from the freshly sliced plant directly to warts or corns. Repeat this application once or twice daily, being careful that the caustic juice does not touch the surrounding skin. Within 3 weeks your warts should have gone.

## GROWING

Cover the bottom of a medium-sized pot with drainage material, then fill with a multipurpose compost. Plant the greater celandine in the centre of the pot in spring and it will grow to fill the pot through the summer. Deadhead to prolong the flowering period. Water regularly and feed weekly.

**Plants you will need**

* *Chelidonium majus* (greater celandine)

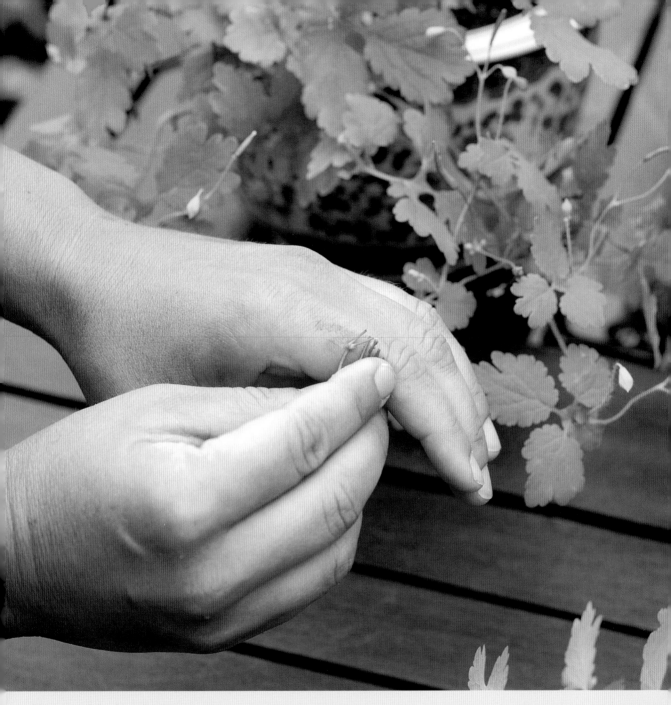

## You could also try...

Applying lemon juice, fresh garlic, the white juice from dandelion stalks or fresh elderberry juice directly to the warts every day ◆ Drinking teas of burdock, dandelion root, echinacea and red clover with a little liquorice to enhance immunity to the wart virus and clear toxins from the system 3–4 times daily ◆ Taking garlic daily, either fresh or as perles ◆ Eating plenty of fresh fruit and vegetables ◆ Taking supplements of cod liver oil, vitamin C, B complex and zinc.

# Reviving eyewash

## For tired eyes and conjunctivitis

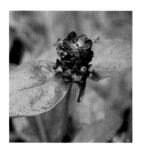

An eyebath made from these herbs is perfect for relieving irritated, inflamed eyes. Plantain cools inflammation; chamomile and marigold (calendula) are antiseptic and anti-inflammatory – excellent for allergic eye problems. Self-heal and coriander reduce swelling and speed healing.

## Ingredients

• 25 g (1 oz) each fresh or 15 g (½ oz) dried marigold (calendula) and chamomile flowers, plantain and coriander leaves, self-heal flowers and leaves
• 600 ml (1 pint) water

Makes 600 ml (1 pint) infusion

## How to make

**1** Place the herbs together in a pan with the water and bring to the boil and remove.
**2** Leave to infuse until lukewarm to cool and then strain.

## How to use

Use sterile eyebath to wash one eye, rinse the eyebath thoroughly and then bathe the other eye. Repeat 3–6 times a day. Store the remainder in the fridge for 2 days, if you wish, but heat it slightly before use.

## GROWING

Cover the bottom of a large square planter with drainage material and top up with a multipurpose compost. Place three marigold (calendula) together in one corner, one plantain in another corner, one self-heal in another corner, four chamomile in the last corner and the coriander in the middle. Deadhead the marigold (calendula) regularly so they keep flowering. Water regularly and feed weekly.

### Plants you will need

• 3 *Calendula officinalis* (marigold)
• 1 *Plantago major/minor/lanceolata* (plantain)
• 1 *Prunella vulgaris* (self-heal)
• 4 *Matricaria recutita* (German chamomile)
• 4 *Coriandrum sativum* (coriander)

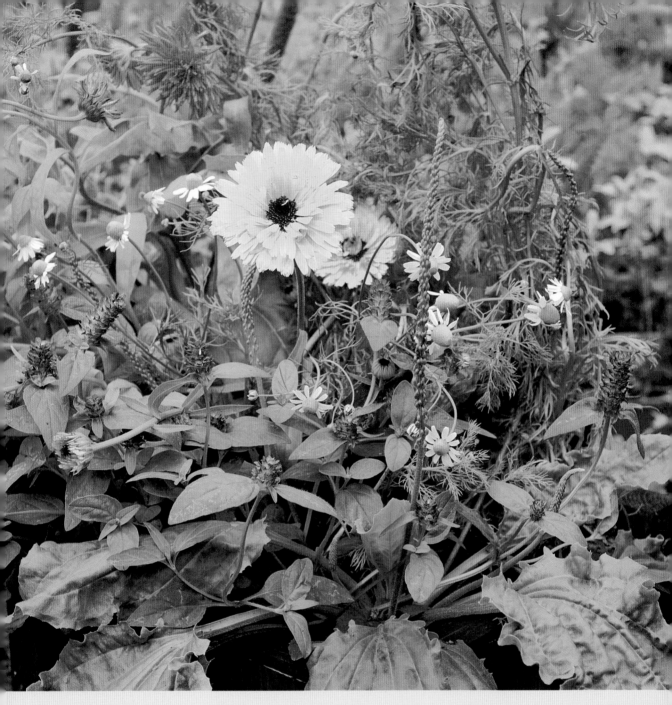

## You could also try...

Wrapping the warmed herbs in a small piece of muslin and placing it over the eye. ♦ Lying quietly for 10–15 minutes 3 times daily ♦ Using black tea to bathe the eyes, or placing a warm chamomile teabag over each eye for 10–15 minutes ♦ Drinking echinacea, chamomile, nettle, lemon balm, red clover or licorice tea to help combat infection ♦ Taking supplements of borage seed or evening primrose oil and vitamin C and B if you suffer from chronic eye problems.

# Stomach settler

## For nausea and vomiting

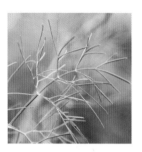

This aromatic drink will help settle nausea and prevent vomiting. Lemon balm and dill calm tension and are excellent for stress-related digestive problems, while peppermint is a digestive remedy, specific for nausea and marshmallow soothes and eases stomach irritation.

## Ingredients

- 3 teaspoons each fresh or 2 teaspoons dried lemon balm, peppermint, dill and marshmallow
- 1¼ litres (2½ pints) boiling water

Makes 1¼ litres (2½ pints) drink

## How to make

**1** Place the herbs in a jug or flask and pour over the boiling water.
**2** Cover and leave to infuse overnight.

## How to use

Sip the infusion throughout the day, whenever you feel the need, until the symptoms have subsided, taking up to 6 cupfuls per day.

### Hints and tips

Peppermint is one of the best remedies for digestive problems, easing spasm and pain, combating infection and inflammation.

## GROWING

Cover the bottom of two medium-sized pots with drainage material and top up with a multipurpose compost. Place the marshmallow plant, which will grow to be quite large. Then plant in two dills next to it. In the second pot, plant a lemon balm and a peppermint and in front of them plant three dills. Water and feed.

**Plants you will need**

- 1 *Althaea officinalis* (marshmallow)
- 5 *Anethum graveolens* (dill)
- 1 *Melissa officinalis* (lemon balm)
- 1 *Mentha piperita* (peppermint)

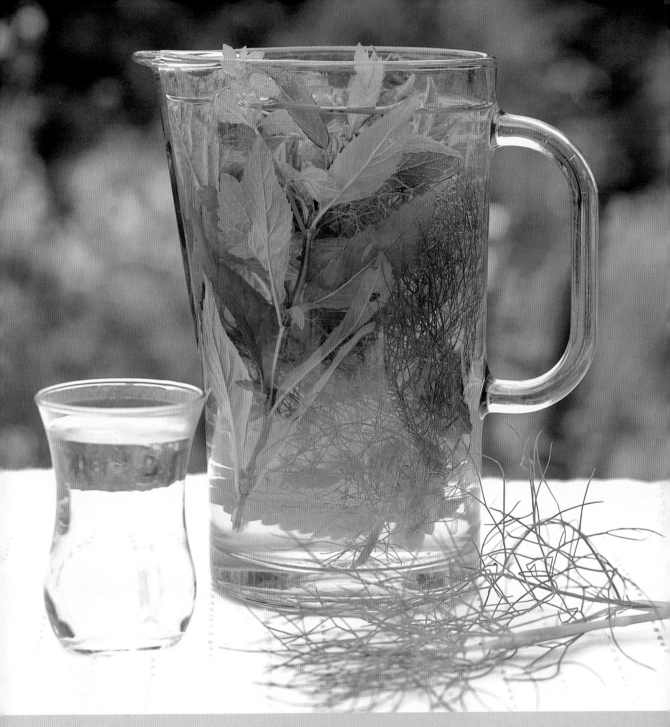

## You could also try...

Sipping fresh ginger tea or simply chewing the root
♦ Adding 1–2 teaspoons of slippery elm to warm rice
milk several times a day ♦ Taking garlic, turmeric,
echinacea, cinnamon, or pau d'arco supplements
every 2 hours in acute infections ♦ Drinking
chamomile, fennel, lavender or thyme tea through
the day ♦ Taking feverfew, wood betony or rosemary
if nausea is associated with headaches or migraine.

# Cooling electuary

## For heartburn and acidity

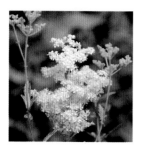

This fragrant array of herbs is a first choice for soothing heartburn and acidity. Meadowsweet is famous for cooling heat and inflammation, while marshmallow is a great demulcent. Lemon balm, chamomile and vervain are calming when heartburn is related to stress.

## Ingredients

- 250 g (9 oz) each fresh or 100 g (3½ oz) dried meadowsweet, marshmallow, lemon balm and chamomile
- 125 g (4½ oz) fresh vervain
- 500 ml (17 fl oz) Manuka or thyme honey

**Makes 500 ml (17 fl oz) electuary**

## How to make

**1** Place the herbs, coarsely chopped, in a clean, sterilized jar. You can use a reusable teabag or tie the herbs into a piece of muslin, if you like.
**2** Cover them with honey and stir well.
**3** Close with an airtight lid, label clearly and leave to macerate for at least 4 weeks. Remove the herbs.
**4** Store in a cool, dark place, preferably the refrigerator.

## How to use

Stir a teaspoonful into a glass of hot water and drink 3–6 times daily.

### Hints and tips

Honey's sweetness brings out the herbs' aromatic flavours. The combination has antimicrobial properties, helping to combat infection.

## GROWING

Cover the bottom of three matching pots with drainage material and top up with a multipurpose compost. Plant the meadowsweet in the large pot, the aloe vera (once all danger of frost has passed) and marshmallow in the medium pot and the lemon balm in the smaller pot. Water regularly and feed weekly.

### Plants you will need

- 1 *Filipendula ulmaria* (meadowsweet)
- 1 *Aloe barbadensis* (aloe vera)
- 1 *Althaea officinalis* (marshmallow)
- 1 *Melissa officinalis* (lemon balm)

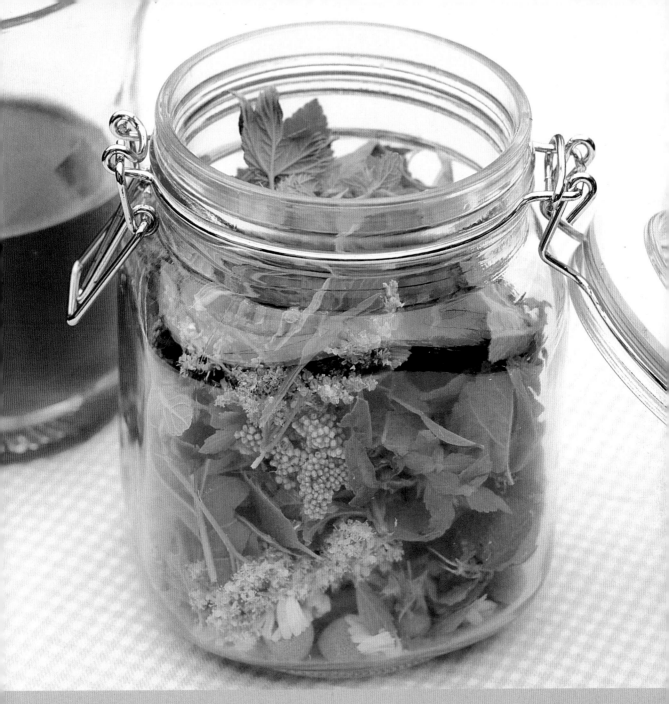

## You could also try...

Avoiding alcohol, chocolate, refined carbohydrates, sugar, tea, coffee, cigarettes, rich, fatty, spicy and acidic foods such as tomatoes and citrus fruits ♦ Avoid getting upset and eating too fast, bending over, sitting hunched up and lying flat in bed ♦ Drinking teas of chamomile, peppermint, dill, basil and licorice to soothe pain and reduce acidity ♦ Eating a gruel made with 1–2 teaspoons of slippery elm powder mixed with warm water 3–4 times daily ♦ Taking 25 ml (1 fl oz) aloe vera juice twice daily.

# Probiotic breakfast

## For dysbiosis

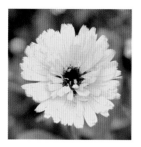

This is a tasty way to start the day. Garlic, calendula, dill, basil and marjoram are excellent for combating pathogenic micro-organisms and are also good digestive herbs, clearing toxins from the digestive tract. Aloe vera is soothing, immune-enhancing and combats dysbiosis.

## Ingredients

- 1 large garlic clove
- 1 tablespoon each fresh dill leaves and marigold (calendula) petals
- 20 ml (1 fl oz) aloe vera juice
- 2 teaspoons each fresh marjoram and thyme
- 1 carton (500 ml/17 fl oz) live yoghurt

**Makes 1 serving**

## How to make

Chop or tear the herbs and add them to a bowl of live yogurt, then stir in the aloe vera juice.

### Did you know?

Probiotic herbs are excellent for supporting beneficial gut bacteria and combating yeasts and bacteria that can take hold after antibiotics or eating badly.

## How to use

Enjoy this yogurt daily. If you are working in close proximity to others you may want to reserve the garlic for weekends and use the other herbs, which are all aromatic and pleasant-tasting You can eat this yoghurt indefinitely.

## GROWING

Cover the bottom of three matching pots with drainage material and top up with a multipurpose compost. Plant the marjoram plants in one corner and place the three marigold (calendula) around it. In the medium-sized pot, plant two dills, the thyme and the garlic. In the third pot plant the aloe vera. Water and feed.

### Plants you will need

- 2 *Origanum marjorana* (marjoram)
- 3 *Calendula officinalis* (marigold)
- 2 *Anethum graveolens* (dill)
- 3 *Thymus vulgaris* (thyme)
- 2 *Allium sativum* (garlic)
- 1 *Aloe barbadensis* (aloe vera)

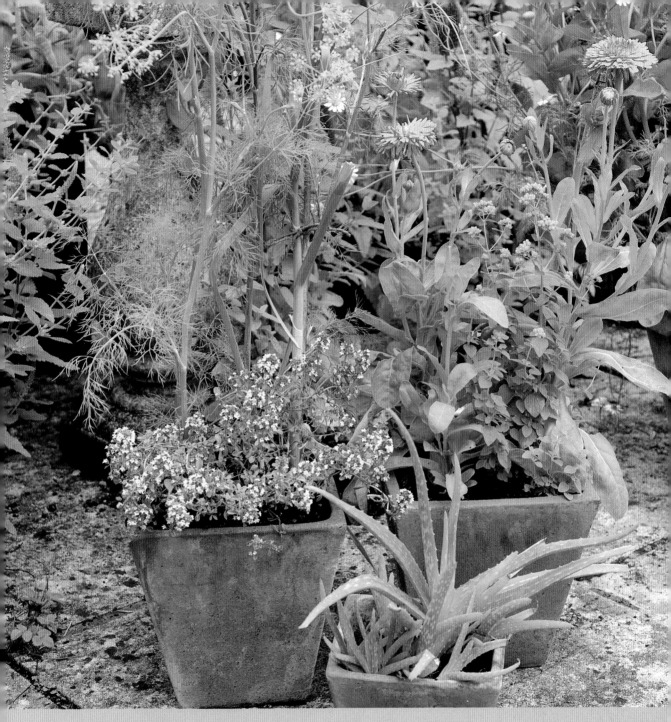

## You could also try...

Drinking teas of fennel, chamomile, thyme, echinacea, and ginger 3–4 times daily. ♦ Adding antimicrobial spices to your cooking daily, including turmeric, cinnamon, ginger and long pepper ♦ Taking supplements of Lactobacillus acidophilus and Bifida bacteria (up to 40 million daily), vitamin C (500 mg daily), caprylic acid (1 g with meals), linseed and evening primrose oil.

# Moving smoothie

## For constipation

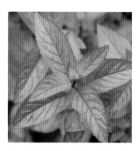

Aloe vera is a panacea for all ills; rich in minerals, vitamins and amino acids, enzymes and other ingredients that help keep bowels regular. Dandelion and flax seed are laxatives, while garlic, thyme, marigold and live yogurt act as probiotics, re-establishing normal bacterial balance.

## Ingredients

- 2 large cloves of garlic
- 2 x 5-cm (2-in) pieces fresh dandelion root, roughly chopped
- 2 teaspoons fresh thyme, peppermint leaves, marigold (calendula) flowers, flax seeds
- 30 ml (1¼ fl oz) aloe vera juice
- 250 ml (9 fl oz) yogurt
- A few slices fresh ginger

**Makes 1 serving**

## How to make

Liquidize the fresh herbs in a blender, with the flax seeds, aloe vera juice, a few slices of fresh ginger and a carton of live organic yoghurt.

## How to use

Drink up and enjoy!

**Did you know?**

It is important to remedy constipation, otherwise toxins formed from re-absorption in the bowel may cause chronic disease.

## GROWING

Cover the bottom of two medium-sized containers with drainage material and top up with a multipurpose compost. Plant the aloe vera and peppermint in one pot and in the other place the thyme near the centre and the dandelions and garlic around it. Water regularly and feed weekly

**Plants you will need**

- 4 *Aloe barbadensis* (aloe vera)
- 1 *Mentha piperita* (peppermint)
- 1 *Thymus vulgaris* (thyme)
- 2 *Taraxacum officinale* (dandelion)
- 2 *Allium sativum* (garlic)

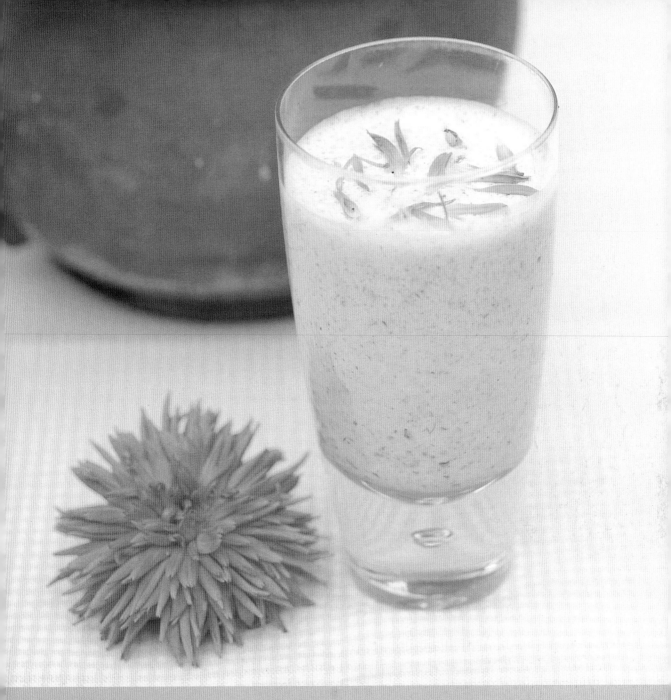

## You could also try...

Avoiding refined foods and eating plenty of fibre in fruit, vegetables and whole grains ♦ Drinking plenty of water ♦ Drinking teas of licorice and burdock 3 times a day ♦ Adding more stimulating laxative herbs such as yellow dock root or senna pods with a little ginger for a week or two ♦ Drinking teas of lemon balm, chamomile, dill, or hops for stress-related problems ♦ Taking supplements of garlic and grapefruit seed extract ♦ Taking 30 minutes of exercise daily.

# Toning tincture

## For diarrhoea

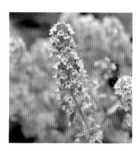

Agrimony is an astringent herb, firming up stools and with analgesic, anti-inflammatory, anti-viral properties. Thyme is excellent for relieving diarrhoea and marshmallow soothes gut lining, while peppermint, lemon balm, dill and chamomile reduce spasm and pain.

## Ingredients

- 250 g (9 oz) each fresh herbs or 100 g (3½ oz) dried dill, peppermint, thyme, agrimony, marshmallow and lemon balm
- 500 ml (17 fl oz) alcohol (vodka, gin or brandy)

Makes 400 ml (14 fl oz) tincture

## How to make

**1** Place the herbs in a large jar and pour over the alcohol.
**2** Place an airtight lid on the jar and leave to macerate, away from direct sunlight, for at least 2 weeks and shake the jar, once daily.
**3** Then squeeze the mixture through a wire sieve, muslin or a wine press to extract the maximum amount of fluid, and discard the herbs.

**4** Transfer the tincture to dark bottles and store in a cool place.

## How to use

Take 1 teaspoon in a little warm water 3–6 times daily.

## GROWING

Cover the bottom of a wooden planter with drainage material and fill with a multipurpose compost. Plant the marshmallow in the centre of the pot. Then in one corner place the thyme, another the agrimony, another the three dills and in the last corner the peppermint and lemon balm. Water regularly and feed weekly.

**Plants you will need**

- 1 *Althaea officinalis* (marshmallow)
- 1 *Thymus vulgaris* (thyme)
- 1 *Agrimonia eupatoria* (agrimony)
- 3 *Anethum graveolens* (dill)
- 1 *Mentha piperita* (peppermint)
- 1 *Melissa officinalis* (lemon balm)

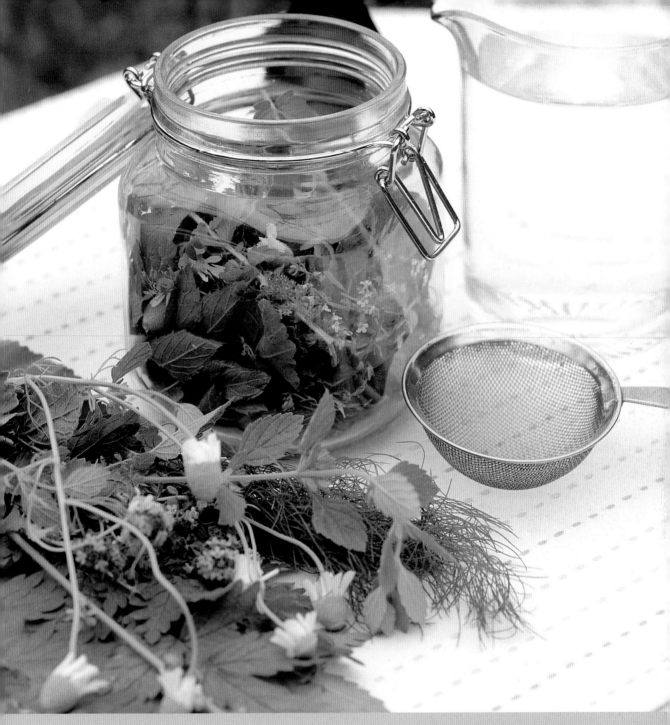

## You could also try...

Drinking plenty of fluids to replace water and electrolytes lost ♦ Drinking teas of cinnamon, raspberry leaf, peppermint, chamomile, lemon balm, ginger, turmeric, coriander or yarrow 3–6 times daily ♦ Taking a gruel made of 1 teaspoon slippery elm powder in a cup of rice milk 3 times daily ♦ Taking supplements of garlic and acidophyllus ♦ Avoiding wheat, dairy and red meat until you feel better.

# Tempting tisane

## For irritable bowel syndrome

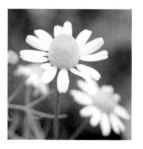

This delightful combination of digestive herbs soothes bowel irritation and inflammation, relaxes tense muscles, relieves pain and helps calm the mind. Chamomile, peppermint, thyme and lemon balm also help combat infection and dysbiosis, possibly underlying IBS.

## Ingredients

- 2 teaspoons each fresh or 1 teaspoon dried chamomile, meadowsweet, peppermint, thyme, agrimony and lemon balm
- 1¼ litres (2½ pints) boiling water

Makes 1¼ litres (2½ pints) infusion

## How to make

**1** Put the herbs in a teapot and cover with the boiling water.
**2** Leave to infuse for 10–15 minutes. Strain.

## How to use

Drink 1 cupful 3–6 times daily and sip slowly.

**Did you know?**

Thyme is rich in antiseptic volatile oils that help re-establish the normal gut flora.

## GROWING

Cover the bottom of three pots with drainage material and top up with a multipurpose compost. In the centre of the large pot plant the peppermint, place the agrimony next to it and three lemon balm at the front. In the medium-sized pot plant the meadowsweet in the centre, the thyme at the front. and the two chamomile in the smaller pot. Water regularly and feed weekly.

**Plants you will need**

- 1 *Mentha piperita* (peppermint)
- 1 *Agrimonia eupatoria* (agrimony)
- 3 *Melissa officinalis* (lemon balm)
- 1 *Filipendula ulmaria* (meadowsweet)
- 1 *Thymus vulgaris* (thyme)
- 2 *Matricaria recutita* (German chamomile) or *Anthemis nobilis/Chamaemelum nobile* (Roman chamomile)

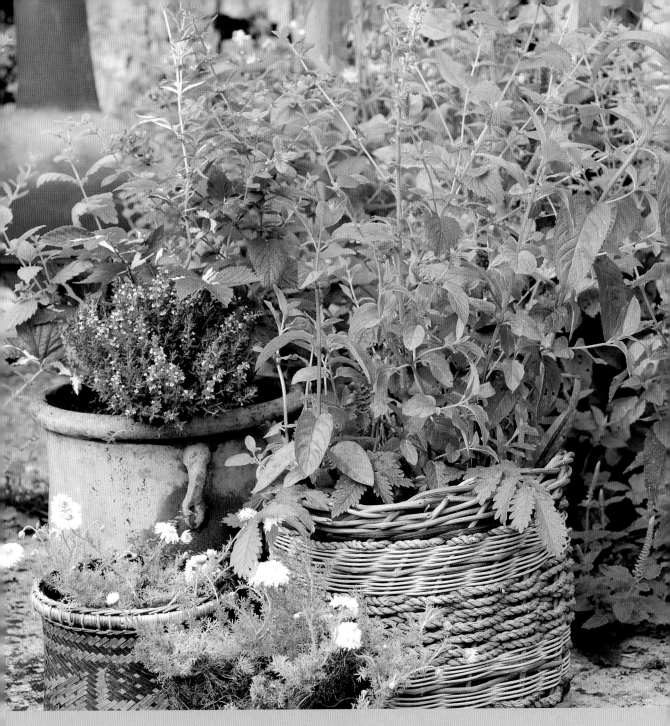

## You could also try...

Temporarily omitting tea, coffee, milk products, sugar, wheat or gluten from your diet ◆ Drinking teas of marshmallow, licorice, vervain, dill or fennel 3–4 times daily ◆ Taking 1–2 teaspoons of slippery elm powder in a little warm rice milk 3–6 times daily ◆ Taking 25 ml (1 fl oz) of aloe vera juice twice daily ◆ Taking supplements of olive leaf, grape seed, garlic and turmeric.

# Summer-time salad

## For obesity

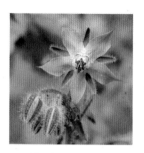

For a great weight-loss salad, try this tasty fusion. Fennel, rocket, nasturtium, coriander and cayenne help increase your metabolism. Dandelion, fennel, coriander and plantain are diuretic, aiding elimination of excess fluid and toxins, while fennel has a reputation for reducing cellulite.

### Ingredients
- 60 g (2½ oz) each young dandelion, plantain and rocket leaves
- Decorate with fennel and coriander leaves, borage leaves and flowers

Serves 2

### How to make

**1** Pick dandelion, plantain, and rocket and put it in a salad bowl.

**2** Garnish with fennel, borage and coriander to taste.

**3** Add nasturtium and a little cayenne pepper, if you want a little more spice, and cucumber if you want a more cooling salad.

**4** Pour over the dressing, made with coconut oil, cider vinegar, garlic and cayenne to stimulate your metabolism.

### How to use
Eat a bowlful and enjoy!

## GROWING

Cover the bottom of a large container with drainage material and top up with a multipurpose compost. Plant the borage in the centre and one nasturtium either side. In the corners of the pot plant the dandelions, a plantain, and two rockets (one in each corner.) In the middle at the back plant the corianders and in the middle at the front plant a cayenne pepper. Next to the cayenne plant the fennel. Water regularly; feed weekly.

**Plants you will need**
- 1 *Borago officinalis* (borage)
- 2 *Tropaeolum majus* (nasturtium)
- 2 *Taraxacum officinale* (dandelion)
- 1 *Plantago major/minor/lanceolata* (plantain)
- 2 *Eruca vesicaria/sativa* (rocket)
- 4 *Coriandrum sativum* (coriander)
- 1 *Capsicum frutescens* (cayenne pepper)
- 3 *Foeniculum vulgare* (fennel)

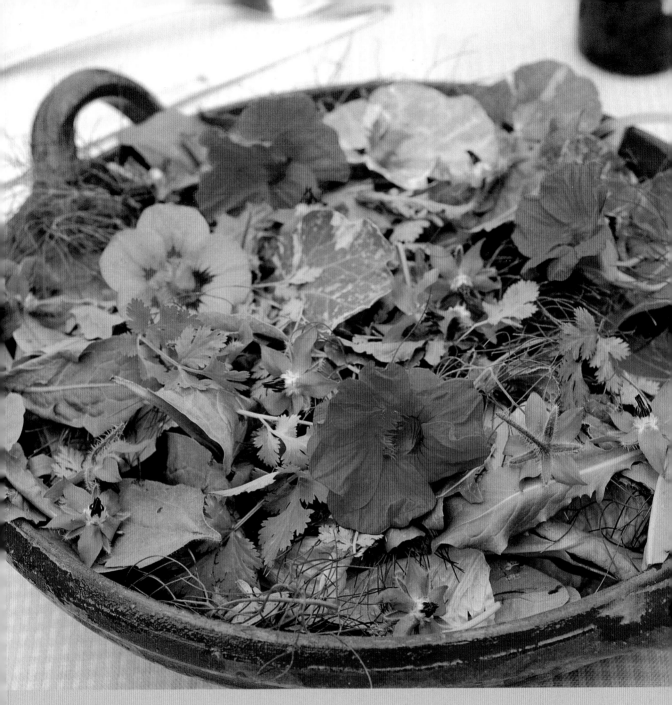

## You could also try...

Teas of plantain, cleavers, chickweed, dandelion leaf, dill, fennel, coriander leaf and parsley 3–4 times daily ◆ Eating plenty of essential fatty acids in oily fish, nuts, seeds, whole grains, evening primrose and flaxseed oil to raise metabolic rate ◆ Trying to lose weight gradually, no more than 1 kg (2 lb) a week ◆ Taking supplements of kelp, guggulu and chromium ◆ Regularly adding spices such as cayenne, garlic, coriander, cumin, ginger, cinnamon, and turmeric to your food.

# Spicy elixir
## For flatulence

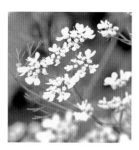

An aromatic elixir prepared from these well-known herbs can be sipped slowly to promote good digestion and prevent and relieve wind. Peppermint, coriander, dill and caraway are excellent digestive and carminative herbs to promote good digestion and relieve wind and bloating.

## Ingredients
+ 500 g (1 ib) honey
+ 500 ml (17 fl oz)brandy
+ 100 g (3½ oz) each fresh or 50 g (2 oz) dried peppermint leaves,
+ 50 g (2 oz) dill, coriander, caraway seeds

Makes 850 ml (28 fl oz) elixir

## How to make

**1** Using equal parts of the herbs place them in a large glass jar and pour over a mixture of honey and brandy.
**2** Add a cinnamon stick and a few slices of fresh ginger, if you like. Press down well so all the herbs are covered.
**3** Leave to infuse for at least 4–6 weeks and then press through a fine mesh strainer or use a wine press.

**4** Label clearly and store in dark bottles in a cool place.

## How to use
Sip half a teaspoon slowly following a meal to promote good digestion and prevent/ relieve wind.

## GROWING

Fill a window box with drainage material and top up with a multipurpose compost. Plant the peppermint in the middle of the pot with the coriander on one side and the caraway on the other. Plant in two dills either side of the peppermint. Water regularly and feed weekly.

**Plants you will need**
+ 1 *Mentha piperita* (peppermint)
+ 3 *Coriandrum sativum* (coriander)
+ 3 *Carum carvi* (caraway)
+ 4 *Anethum graveolens* (dill)

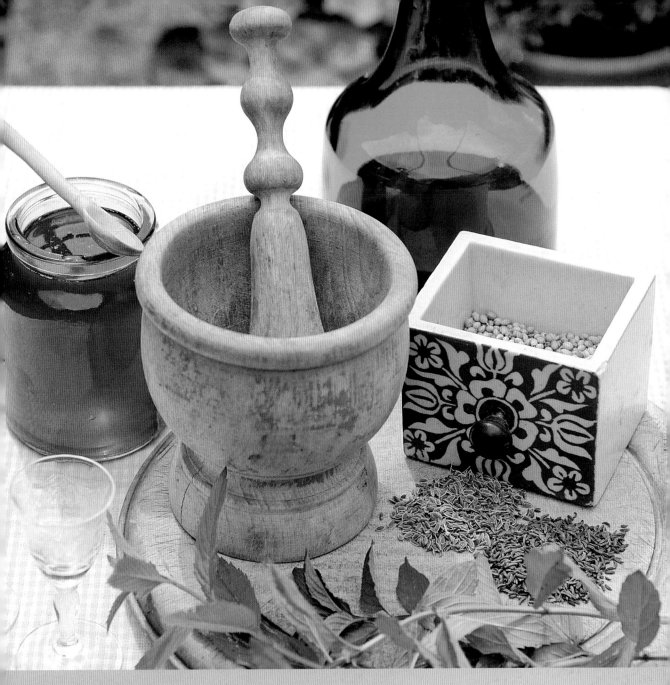

## You could also try...

Drinking teas of fennel, dill, rosemary, peppermint, ginger, cinnamon, lemon balm and chamomile. ♦ Chewing cumin, coriander, cardamom, fennel and dill seeds before and after meals. ♦ Adding mild spices to cooking to enhance digestion ♦ Drinking ginger tea regularly ♦ Taking supplements of acidophyllus, garlic, olive leaf, goldenseal, turmeric, and oregano oil for dysbiosis ♦ Eating slowly when relaxed and not late at night ♦ Exercising to enhance digestion ♦ Eliminating wheat and dairy from the diet ♦ Gently massaging the abdomen using dilute oils of cinnamon, ginger, cloves or peppermint.

# Refreshing mouthwash
## For mouth and gum problems

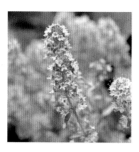

Good oral hygiene and immunity will keep mouth and gum problems at bay. Antiseptic sage, thyme and calendula are excellent for prevention and treatment. They contain tannins that help to heal sore gums and thyme contains thymol, an antiseptic essential oil to help combat infection.

## Ingredients
+ 1 teaspoon each fresh or ½ teaspoon dried of sage, calendula, thyme
+ 200 ml (7 fl oz) boiling water

Makes 200 ml (7 fl oz) mouthwash

## How to make
Steep the herbs, covered in a cup of boiling water for 30 minutes. Strain.

### Did you know?
Marigold (calendula) flowers are an excellent antibacterial, antiviral and antifungal for all kinds of infections in the mouth.

## How to use
Rinse your mouth with the infusion morning and night. You can also dip your dental floss in the tea before using it. Use frequently to calm inflammation associated with gingivitis and to strengthen the gums.

## GROWING

Cover the bottom of a medium container with drainage material and top up with a multipurpose compost. Place the sage in the front left corner and the thyme in the back right corner and then plant in three marigolds (calendulas) diagonally across the box. Deadhead the marigold (calendula) so that they repeat flower. Water regularly and feed weekly.

### Plants you will need
+ 1 *Salvia officinalis* (sage)
+ 1 *Thymus vulgaris* (thyme)
+ 3 *Calendula officinalis* (marigold)

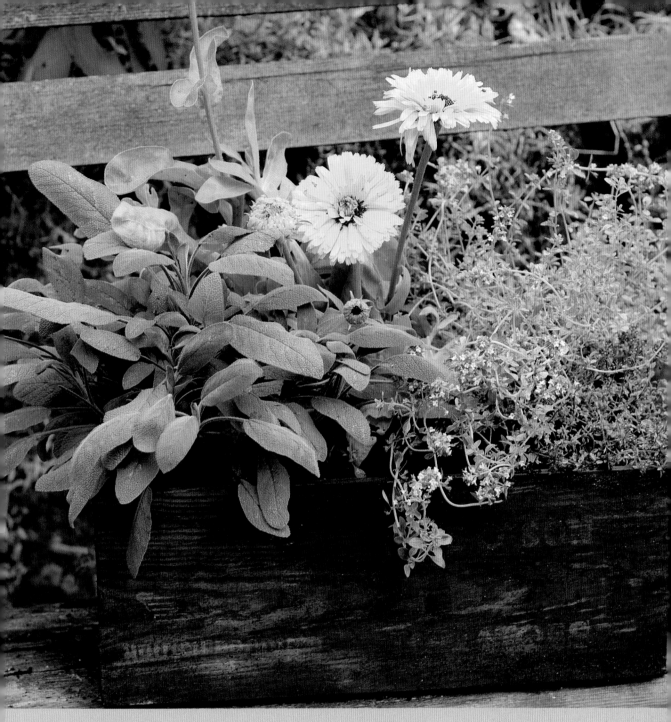

## You could also try...

Rinsing the mouth regularly with antiseptic infusions of cat's claw, peppermint, chamomile, goldenseal, agrimony or myrrh ✦ Drinking teas of the herbs to enhance immunity ✦ Taking supplements of vitamin C and bioflavonoids ✦ Taking supplements of antioxidant herbs bilberry, hawthorn, cat's claw, self-heal, grape seed and oregano to protect blood vessels from free radical damage ✦ Flossing daily.

# Brilliant brain tonic

## For poor memory and concentration

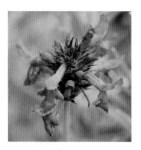

This exquisitely refreshing drink acts as a veritable brain tonic. Rosemary, thyme and peppermint enliven the mind, while wood betony sends blood to the brain. Gotu kola stimulates blood flow to the head, clearing the mind, enhancing concentration and increasing creativity.

## Ingredients

- 60 g (2½ oz) each fresh or 30 g (1 oz) dried rosemary, thyme, gotu kola, peppermint, wood betony
- 600 ml (1 pint) water
- 500 g (1 lb) sugar
- 30 ml (1 fl oz) brandy (optional)

**Makes 650 ml (21 fl oz) tonic**

## How to make

**1** Pour the boiling water over the herbs.
**2** Leave to infuse overnight, then strain through a fine mesh sieve or muslin into a jug and press as much residual water from the herb mixture before discarding it.
**3** Mix the sugar into the infusion in a pan and heat it until the sugar has dissolved and the mixture has started to thicken, stirring frequently. If desired, add 5 per cent brandy to preserve the syrup.
**4** Store in sterilized dark bottles, clearly labelled and keep in a cool place, preferably the refrigerator, for up to 6 months.

## How to use

Take 2 teaspoons 3–4 times daily, over several weeks, for good effect.

## GROWING

Cover the bottom of two wooden boxes with drainage material and top up with multipurpose compost. Plant the rosemary, gotu kola and wood betony in one pot and the thyme and peppermint in the other. Do not let the gotu kola pot dry out as it loves damp, but do not waterlog as rosemary does not! Water regularly and feed weekly.

**Plants you will need**

- 1 *Rosmarinus officinalis* (rosemary)
- 1 *Centella/Hydrocotyle asiatica* (gotu kola)
- 1 *Stachys betonica* (wood betony)
- 1 *Thymus vulgaris* (thyme)
- 1 *Mentha piperita* (peppermint)

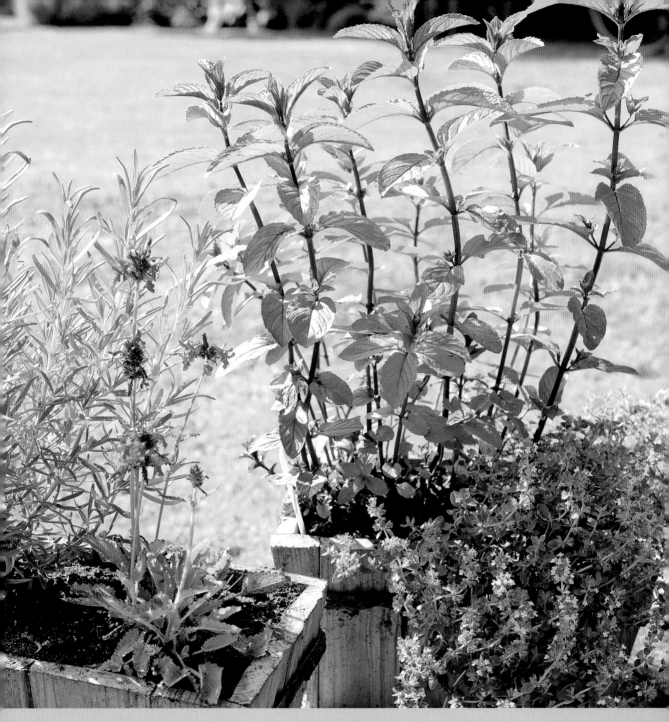

## You could also try...

Drinking teas of gotu kola, periwinkle and ginkgo to increase flow of blood and nutrients to the brain ◆ Taking supplements of rhodiola, B vitamins, lecithin, antioxidant vitamins A, C and E, co-enzyme Q 10 and essential fatty acids ◆ Taking ginseng, hawthorn, ashwagandha, thyme, St John's wort, or schizandra to protect the brain cells by preventing damage from free radicals.

# Pain-relief compress

## For headaches and migraine

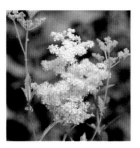

Rosemary helps tense muscles that bring on stress headaches to soften and relax, while meadowsweet is ideal for relieving pain. Feverfew is famed for helping intractable headaches, bringing blood to the head, while refreshing peppermint makes a great analgesic.

## Ingredients

- 30 g (1 oz) each fresh or 15 g (½ oz) dried rosemary, peppermint, feverfew, meadowsweet
- 250 ml (9 fl oz) white vinegar

Makes 250 ml (9 fl oz) jar

## How to make

**1** Fill the jar with the herbs.
**2** Cover with the vinegar and leave on a sunny windowsill for 2–3 weeks.
**3** Strain into a clean, dark bottle and seal.

## How to use

When you have a headache, pour some of the vinegar into a bowl and soak a clean flannel in it, wring out and apply to the forehead. Repeat as necessary. You can also chill the bowl of vinegar in the fridge, which will help if your headaches are relieved by cold temperatures.

### Hints and tips

Rosemary relieves headaches of all kinds, whether from stress, poor circulation, muscle tension or the excesses of the night before.

## GROWING

Cover the bottom of an assortment of pots with drainage material and top up with multipurpose compost. Plant each herb in an individual pot and group the pots together to look appealing. Water regularly and feed weekly.

**Plants you will need**

- 1 *Filipendula ulmaria* (meadowsweet)
- 1 *Rosmarinus officinalis* (rosemary)
- 1 *Chrysanthemum parthenium/Tanacetum parthenium* (feverfew)
- 1 *Mentha piperita* (peppermint)

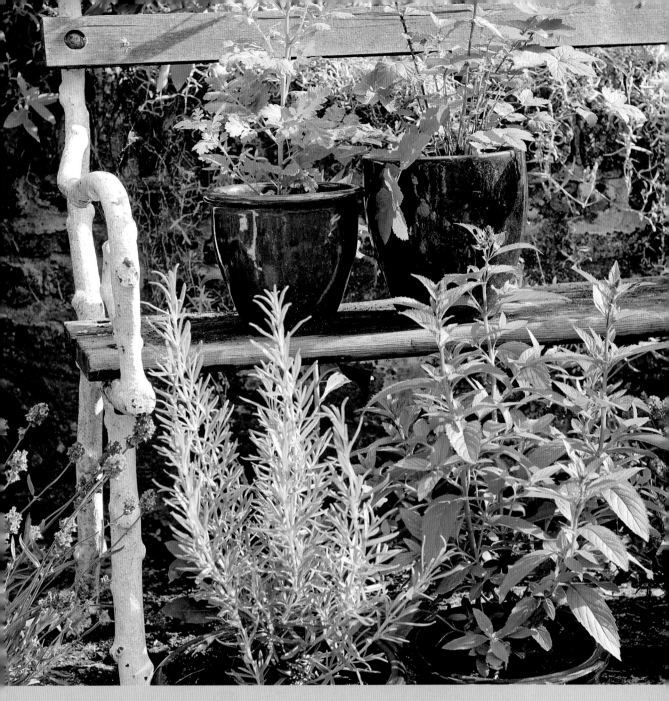

## You could also try...

Using the same herbs for tea to drink 3–6 times daily or foot baths 3 times daily for 10 minutes ♦ Drinking teas of lemon balm, wood betony, gotu kola, milk thistle and ginkgo 3–4 times daily as a preventative ♦ Drinking teas of pain-killing herbs passionflower, California poppy, hops, skullcap, chamomile or vervain up to every hour or two during a headache ♦ Inhaling lavender, peppermint or rosemary oils or massaging them into the temples ♦ Massaging the head, neck and feet with gotu kola oil.

# De-stressing soak

## For tension and anxiety

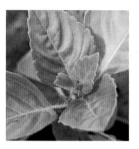

On a stressful day you might feel the need to sip a calming tea or soak in a bath to release tense muscles and calm anxious thoughts. This combination of relaxing herbs not only looks, tastes and smells inviting, but also relaxes tense muscles, calms nerves and soothes troubles away.

## Ingredients

+ 100 g (3½ oz) each fresh or 50 g (2 oz) dried skullcap, chamomile, vervain, lemon balm, holy basil

**Makes enough for 1 bath**

## How to make

Place 1 or 2 handfuls of the herbs in a piece of muslin or cotton and tie a string around the top to close the opening. Make sure that the string is long enough so that the bag soaks in the water once the bath is filled.

## How to use

Tie the bag to the hot bath tap and soak for 15–30 minutes, or until you feel more relaxed.

### Did you know?

Lemon balm used to be known as 'scholar's herb' as it calms anxiety and promotes memory and concentration at the same time.

## GROWING

Cover the bottom of a large pot with drainage material and top up with multipurpose compost. Plant the lemon balm in the centre, the vervain on one side and Virginian skullcap on the other. Then put two chamomiles in the back and two at the front with the holy basil. Water regularly and feed weekly.

**Plants you will need**

+ 1 *Melissa officinalis* (lemon balm)
+ 1 *Verbena officinalis* (vervain)
+ 1 *Scutellaria lateriflora* (Virginian skullcap)
+ 4 *Matricaria recutita* (German chamomile) or *Anthemis nobilis/Chamamaelum nobile* (Roman chamomile)
+ 1 *Ocimum sanctum* (holy basil)

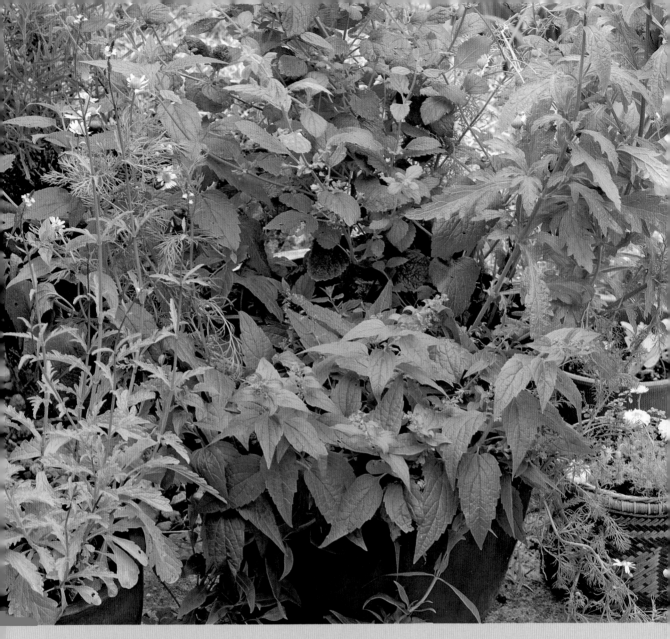

## You could also try...

Drinking teas of the herbs (see left) 3–6 times a day ♦ Drinking teas of other calming herbs such as passionflower, holy basil, California poppy, rose, motherwort, lavender, limeflower, and hops every hour or two, if necessary ♦ Taking adaptogens such as ginseng, ashwagandha, gotu kola, schizandra, wild asparagus or licorice to strengthen the nerves and increase resilience to stress ♦ Having a relaxing massage with oils of holy basil, nutmeg, lavender, rosemary, rose or chamomile in a base of sesame oil ♦ Taking regular aerobic exercise to stimulate secretion of endorphins and increase resilience to stress. ♦ Practising meditation and breathing exercises ♦ Avoiding caffeine, sugar, alcohol and junk foods ♦ Taking supplements of calcium, magnesium and vitamin-B complex.

# Uplifting tisane
## For depression

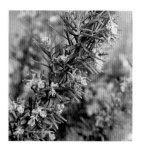

When you are feeling low there's herbal help at hand from pots right outside your door. St John's wort can dispel the blues and borage supports the adrenal glands, lifting the spirits. The lemony scent of lemon balm with rosemary and clary sage can make you feel better straight away.

## Ingredients

♦ 2 teaspoons each fresh or 1 teaspoon dried lemon balm, clary sage, rosemary, St John's wort, borage, lavender
♦ 1¼ litre (2½ pints) boiling water

Makes 1¼ litre (2½ pints)

## How to make

**1** Place the herbs in a teapot and pour over boiling water.
**2** Leave to infuse for 10–15 minutes.

## How to use

Drink a cupful 3–6 times daily. For best effects you may need to take these herbs over several weeks.

### Please note

It is important not to drink alcohol when taking clary sage and observe the contraindications for St John's wort (see page 129).

## GROWING

Cover the bottom of four matching pots with drainage material and top up with multipurpose compost. In the largest pot place the St John's wort on one side and the rosemary on the other. Place the clary sage in front. Plant the borage in another and the lavender and lemon balm in the last. Water regularly and feed weekly.

### Plants you will need

♦ 1 *Hypericum perforatum* (St John's wort)
♦ 1 *Rosmarinus officinalis* (rosemary)
♦ 2 *Salvia sclarea* (clary sage)
♦ 1 *Borago officinalis* (borage)
♦ 1 *Lavandula officinalis* (lavender)
♦ 1 *Melissa officinalis* (lemon balm)

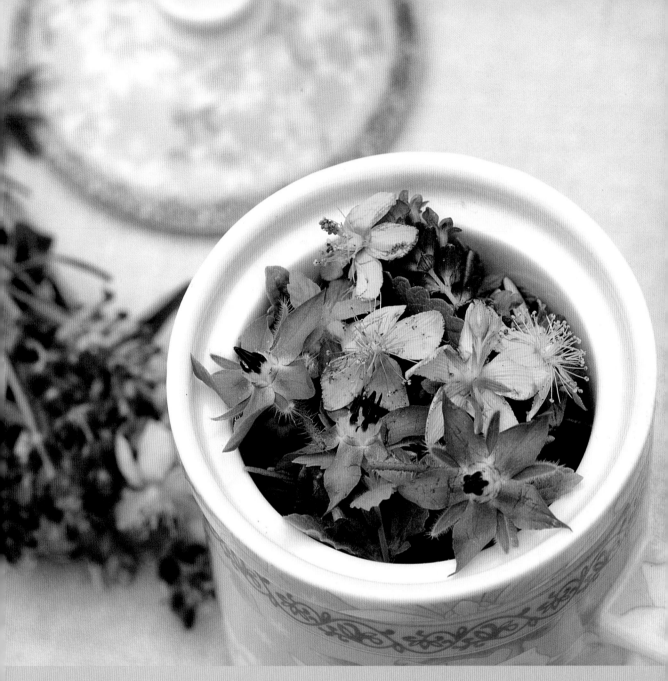

## You could also try...

Drinking teas of mood-elevating herbs, wild oats, vervain, skullcap, basil or wood betony 3–6 times daily ◆ Taking supplements of adaptogen herbs ginkgo, Siberian ginseng, rhodiola, gotu kola or licorice to increase resilience to stress ◆ Adding essential oils of lavender, rosemary, chamomile, bergamot, or rose to baths/massage oils ◆ Taking rose, wild asparagus, vitex, evening primrose or black cohosh for depression related to PMS or the menopause ◆ Taking regular exercise ◆ Avoiding caffeine, alcohol and junk foods ◆ Taking supplements of omega-3, vitamin C, B complex and magnesium.

# Invigorating foot bath

## For tiredness and exhaustion

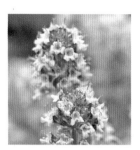

These enlivening herbs provide ingredients for an invigorating foot bath should exhaustion strike. Rosemary and holy basil are rich in antioxidants, increase resilience to stress and stimulate the mind; vervain and holy basil strengthen nerves. Borage is good for adrenal exhaustion.

## Ingredients

- 100 g (3½ oz) each fresh or 50 g (2 oz) dried rosemary, vervain, holy basil, thyme, borage
- 1¼ litres (2½ pints) water

Makes 1¼ litres (2½ pints) footbath

## How to make

**1** Place the herbs in a teapot.
**2** Pour over boiling water and leave to infuse for about half an hour.

### Hints and tips

Vervain is a great tonic for the nervous system and supports the body during stressful times.

## How to use

Pour into a bowl that is large enough for your feet, check that the temperature is right and then soak your feet for 15–30 minutes twice a day, or when you feel the need for renewed energy.

## GROWING

In four large pots, cover the bottoms with drainage material and fill with a multipurpose compost. In the first pot plant the borage in the middle and surround with four basils. In the second pot plant the vervain, in the third pot plant the rosemary and in the fourth pot plant the thyme. Water regularly and feed weekly.

### Plants you will need

- 1 *Borago officinalis* (borage)
- 4 *Ocimum sanctum* (holy basil)
- 1 *Verbena officinalis* (vervain)
- 1 *Rosmarinus officinalis* (rosemary)
- 1 *Thymus vulgaris* (thyme)

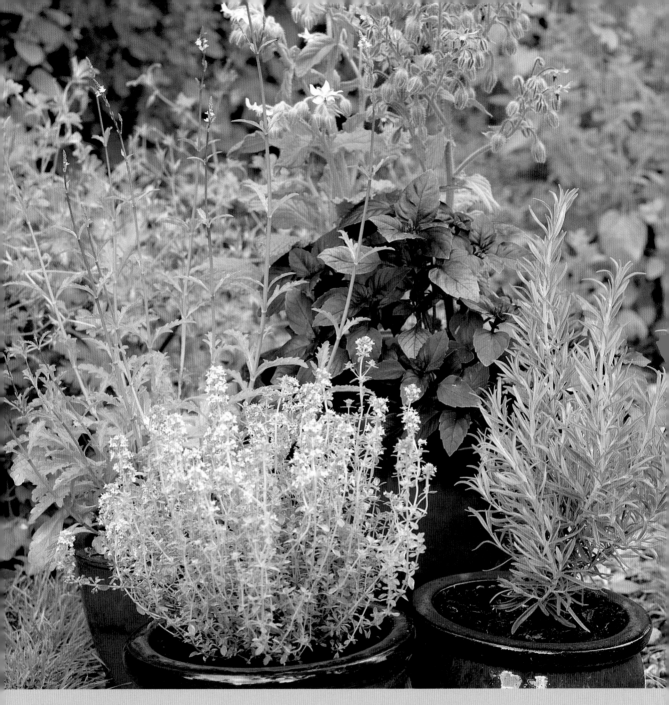

## You could also try...

Eating plenty of whole grains, fruits, vegetables, protein and essential fatty acids ♦ Drinking teas of the herbs (see left) 3–6 times daily ♦ Drinking teas of rejuvenating herbs such as wild oats, ginseng, gotu kola, ashwagandha, vervain or licorice 3–4 times daily ♦ Avoiding coffee, alcohol, sugar and junk foods Taking dandelion, burdock, red clover, or nettles if you are run down from illness or long-term drug therapy ♦ Taking supplements of vitamin C, co-enzyme Q10, magnesium, B complex and zinc.

# Herb sleep pillow

## For insomnia

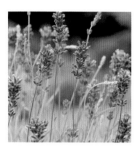

Before you rush to the doctor for sleeping pills, try some natural treatments first. The delicately scented herbs in this recipe have soporific qualities that promote relaxing sleep. Their fragrant essential oils are carried straight to the brain, calming tension and promoting sleep.

## Ingredients

♦ 75 g (3 oz) each dried lavender and chamomile flowers, holy basil, California poppy, lemon balm leaves
♦ oblong of cotton fabric large enough to make a small pillow

**Makes 1 herb pillow**

## How to make

**1** Mix the herbs together in a bowl, add a few drops of lavender oil, if you wish,
**2** Stitch up 3 sides of the fabric oblong. Stuff the herbs into the bag and stitch up the remaining opening, to make a small pillow.

## How to use

Use at the side of your usual pillow to promote restful sleep and a clear head. You could also place the herbs loose in a bowl by your bedside.

### Hints and tips
California poppy is an excellent herb for insomnia; gentle and non-addictive.

## GROWING

Sow the California poppy seeds in spring. In early summer cover the bottom of two large pots with drainage material and top up with multipurpose compost. Place the lavender in one of the pots and the lemon balm, holy basil and chamomile in the other pot. Water regularly and feed weekly.

### Plants you will need

♦ 1 *Eschscholzia californica* (California poppy)
♦ 1 *Lavandula officinalis* (lavender)
♦ 1 *Melissa officinalis* (lemon balm)
♦ 1 *Ocimum sanctum* (holy basil)
♦ 1 *Matricaria recutita* (German chamomile) or *Anthemis nobilis/Chamaemelum nobile* (Roman chamomile)

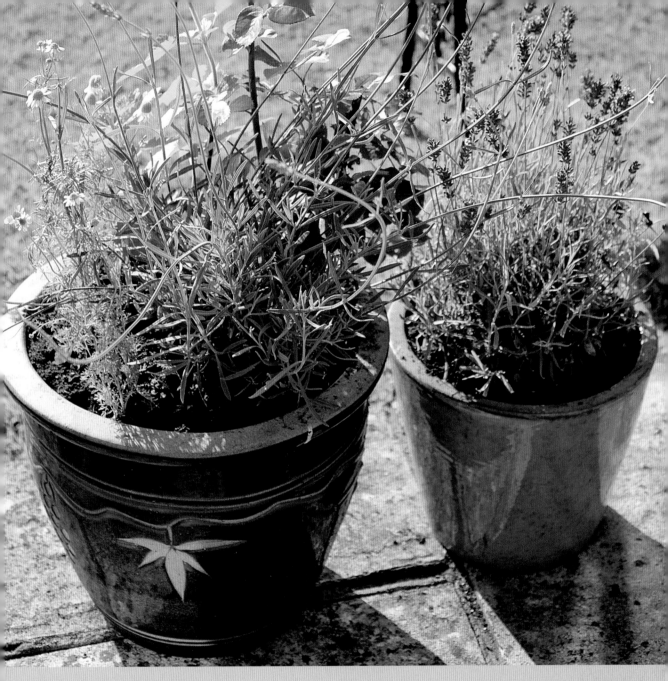

## You could also try...

Eating plenty of oats, whole grains, fresh fruit and vegetables, nuts and seeds ♦ Avoiding stimulants including sugar, sweets, caffeine and smoking, especially near bedtime ♦ Avoiding stimulating the brain at night, or eating a large meal near bedtime ♦ Drinking hot milk with nutmeg and honey, or lemon balm, lavender, chamomile or limeflower tea before bed ♦ Taking supplements of valerian, hops and passionflower before bed ♦ Taking supplements of B complex, calcium and magnesium, 5-HTP and inositol ♦ Taking regular exercise ♦ Having a warm sesame oil massage followed by a bath before bed.

# Healing tisane

## For arthritis and gout

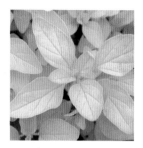

A tisane of marjoram, nettles, gotu kola and feverfew can make a tea and a foot bath. Gotu kola and feverfew are wonderful anti-inflammatories, nettles are packed with nutrients, improve circulation and help clear toxins. Marjoram improves circulation and helps fight ageing.

## Ingredients

- 2 teaspoons each fresh or 1 teaspoon dried marjoram, nettle, gotu kola and feverfew leaves
- 1¼ litres (2½ pints) boiling water

Makes 1¼ litres (2½ pints) tisane

## How to make

Place the herbs in a teapot and pour on boiling water and leave to infuse for 10–15 minutes.

**Did you know?**

Marjoram's diuretic properties help relieve fluid retention and enhance elimination of toxins that can contribute to arthritis and gout.

## How to use

Drink 1 cupful 3 times daily before meals. A stronger tisane left to infuse for 30 minutes or more can be poured into a bowl and used as a warm foot bath at night.

## GROWING

Fill three medium-sized planters with a multipurpose compost. Plant the feverfew in one pot, the gotu kola and golden marjoram in another and nettle in the other. Pick the nettle leaves frequently to promote the growth of more young leaves and prevent it going to seed. Water regularly and feed weekly.

**Plants you will need**

- 2 *Centella/Hydrocotyle asiatica* (gotu kola)
- 1 *Chrysanthemum parthenium/Tanacetum parthenium* (feverfew)
- 1 *Origanum majorana* (marjoram)
- 1 *Urtica dioica* (nettle)

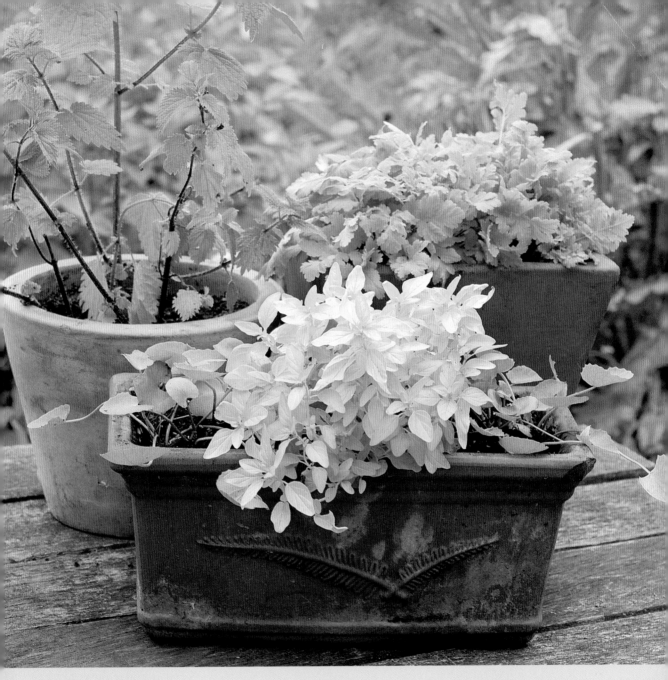

## You could also try...

Supplements of evening primrose oil, glucosamine sulphate, MSM, omega-3 oils and selenium to promote repair of cartilage ♦ Taking supplements of turmeric, boswellia, devil's claw, black cohosh, licorice, ashwagandha, gotu kola, burdock, nettles, or echinacea ♦ Drinking a cup of ginger tea 3 times daily ♦ Avoiding excess fatty foods, red meat, nightshades (potatoes, peppers, aubergines and tomatoes), cheese, citrus fruits and alcohol ♦ Massaging with liniments with essential oils of rosemary or marjoram and a few drops of cayenne tincture to increase circulation to the joint and reduce pain.

# Magic massage oil

## For muscular aches and pains

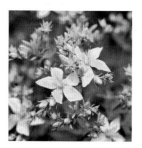

Massaging aching muscles with rosemary oil, St John's wort and chamomile will help to ease muscle spasm. Rosemary stimulates blood flow, clears toxins and relieves pain, St John's wort is for muscle tension and nerve pain, while chamomile is analgesic and anti-inflammatory.

## Ingredients

- 100 g (3½ oz) each fresh or 50 g (2 oz) dried rosemary leaves, chamomile and St John's wort flowers
- 250 ml (9 fl oz) cold-pressed sesame, almond or olive oil

Makes 250 ml (9 fl oz) oil

## How to make

**1** Place freshly crushed herbs in a clear glass jar and cover them with the oil.
**2** Place the jar, tightly lidded, in a sunny place for 2–3 weeks.
**3** Strain the oil through a fine mesh sieve or muslin, pressing as much oil as you can and discard the flowers.
**4** Pour the oil into a bottle to store. Label clearly.

## How to use

Massage the warmed oil into the painful muscles 2 or 3 times daily until pain subsides. Massage is best followed by a hot bath or shower.

## GROWING

Fill the bottom of a large circular pot with drainage material and top up with a multipurpose compost. Place the rosemary in the centre, the St John's wort at the back and the chamomiles in front. Water regularly and feed weekly.

**Plants you will need**

- 1 *Rosmarinus officinalis* (rosemary)
- 1 *Hypericum perforatum* (St John's wort)
- 2 *Matricaria recutita* (German chamomile) or *Anthemis nobilis/Chamaemelum nobile* (Roman chamomile)

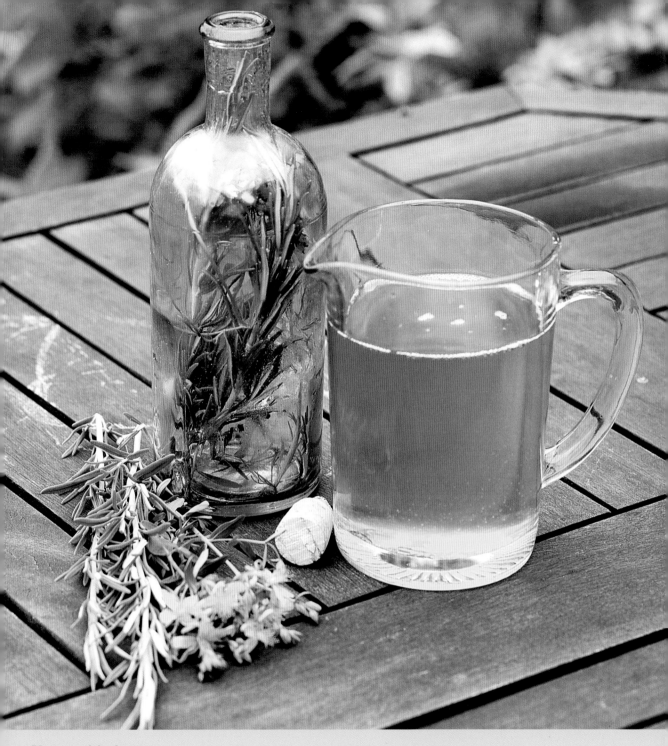

## You could also try...

Using marjoram, thyme, basil, lavender or ginger in massage oils and liniments ♦ Drinking teas of muscle-relaxing and pain-relieving herbs such as rosemary, thyme, chamomile, ginger, lavender, basil, skullcap and ashwagandha 3–4 times a day ♦ Taking supplements of B complex, calcium and magnesium.

# Muscle-ease liniment

## For cramp relief

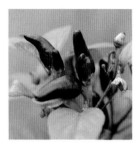

This eye-catching arrangement, with its purple thyme flowers and peppers will ease the muscular spasm that causes cramp. Together the cayenne, rosemary and thyme relax spasm and ease pain. Massaging aids the absorption of the remedy.

## Ingredients

- 1 small cayenne pepper
- 150 g (5½ oz) each fresh or 75 g (3 oz) dried rosemary and thyme sprigs
- 100 ml (3½ fl oz) unrefined sesame oil
- 250 ml (9 fl oz) alcohol, such as vodka or brandy

Makes 350 ml (11 fl oz) liniment

## How to make

**1** Chop the herbs coarsely and place in the jar.
**2** Pour over the alcohol to cover the herbs, cover with an airtight lid and store in a warm, dark place for 7–10 days, shaking well at least once a day.
**3** Strain the mixture through muslin or a strainer, squeezing the herbs to extract as much of the liquid as possible.

**4** Measure the liquid and add the sesame oil.
**5** Add a few drops of essential oil of rosemary for a more penetrating smell and effect. Pour it into a glass bottle and label.

## How to use

Massage your calves with the liniment nightly before bed.

## GROWING

Place drainage material in the base of a large pot and fill with multipurpose compost. Plant the rosemary in the centre, the thymes in the front and the cayenne at the back, once all danger of frosts has passed. Be careful not to overwater as thyme and rosemary are Mediterranean herbs that flourish in dry ground.

### Plants you will need

- 1 *Rosmarinus officinalis* (rosemary)
- 2 *Thymus vulgaris* (thyme)
- 1 *Capsicum frutescens* (cayenne pepper)

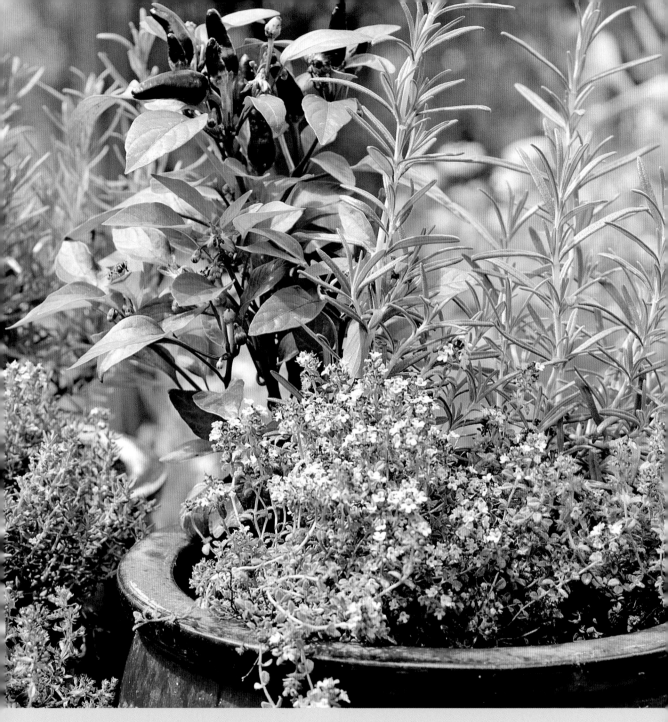

## You could also try...

Drinking plenty of fluid ♦ Drinking teas to increase blood flow to muscles, such as ginger, gotu kola, turmeric, ginkgo, hawthorn, cinnamon, coriander seed or cayenne 3–4 times daily ♦ Eating garlic and adding calcium-rich herbs to your diet, including nettles, dill, wild oats, celery seed, meadowsweet, borage, and dandelion leaves ♦ Taking supplements of vitamins B, D and C, calcium and magnesium.

# Herbal tincture

## For high blood pressure

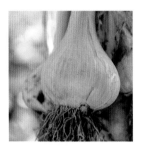

Motherwort, gotu kola and yarrow relax and dilate the arteries while lemon balm is an antioxidant herb, helping to prevent artery damage and reducing risk of heart attack and stroke. Dandelion helps relieve artery pressure while garlic is famous for its ability to open the arteries.

## Ingredients

- 250 g (9 oz) each fresh or 100 g (3½ oz) dried motherwort, gotu kola, yarrow, lemon balm, dandelion leaf
- 2 cloves garlic
- 500 ml (17 fl oz) alcohol (vodka, gin or brandy)

Makes 400 ml (14 fl oz) tincture

## How to make

**1** Place the herbs in a large jar and pour over the alcohol.
**2** Place an airtight lid on the jar and leave to macerate away from direct sunlight for at least a fortnight and shake the jar once daily.
**3** Then squeeze the mixture through a sieve, muslin or a wine press to extract the maximum amount of fluid and discard the herb.

**4** Transfer the tincture to a dark bottle, label clearly and store in a cool place.

## How to use

Take 1 teaspoon in a little water 3 times daily before meals. This may need to be taken over several weeks for good effect.

## GROWING

Cover the bottom of a set of matching pots with drainage material and top up with a multipurpose compost. Plant the lemon balm in the centre of the largest pot, place the yarrow behind it and the garlic on either side. Plant the motherwort in the centre of the second pot, with gotu kola in the front. Plant the dandelions in the third pot. Water everything regularly and feed weekly.

### Plants you will need

- 1 *Melissa officinalis* (lemon balm)
- 1 *Achillea millefolium* (yarrow)
- 2 *Allium sativum* (garlic)
- 1 *Leonurus cardiaca* (motherwort)
- 1 *Centella/Hydrocotyle asiatica* (gotu kola)
- 3 *Taraxacum officinale* (dandelion)

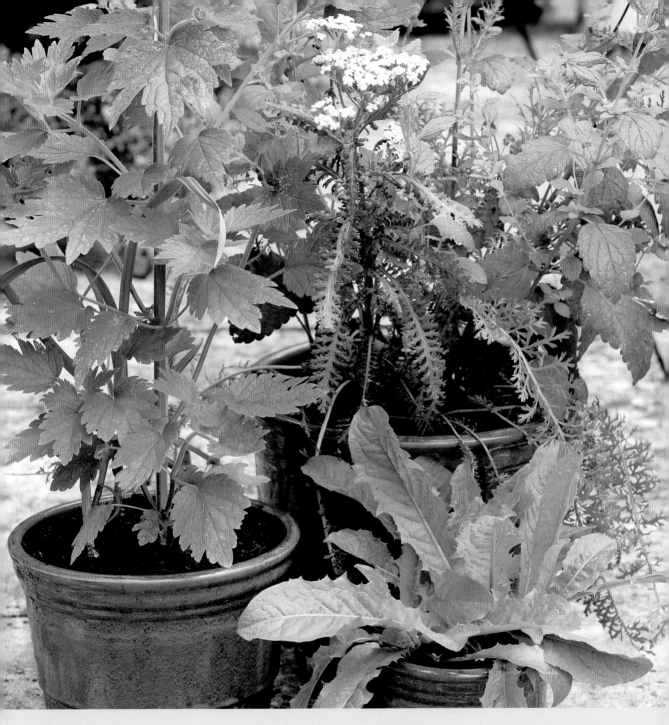

## You could also try...

Drinking anti-hypertensive teas of hawthorn, limeflowers, ginkgo, or valerian 3–4 times daily ◆ Eating antioxidant blueberries and elderberries regularly ◆ Drinking teas of chamomile, passionflower, or skullcap to reduce tension and anxiety ◆ Eating a largely vegetarian diet with plenty of cold-pressed vegetable oils ◆ Avoiding tea, coffee, alcohol and smoking ◆ Taking regular aerobic exercise.

# Herb-infused flaxseed oil

## For high cholesterol

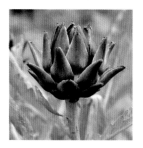

This health-giving oil makes an excellent salad dressing, lowering cholesterol and blood pressure. Garlic also lowers blood cholesterol, helping prevent heart attacks. Calendula and artichoke help liver metabolism of cholesterol, while marjoram and basil strengthen blood vessels.

## Ingredients

+ 1 litre (1¾ pint) flaxseed oil
+ 1 bulb garlic
+ 3 artichoke leaves
+ 400 g (14 oz) each fresh or 200 g (7 oz) dried marigold (calendula) flowers, marjoram leaves, basil flowers and leaves

**Makes 1 litre
(1¾ pint) oil**

## How to make

**1** Bruise the flowers and leaves and place them in a large jar, using as many as you need to almost fill the jar.
**2** Pour over enough oil to cover the herbs and leave to infuse on a sunny windowsill for 2–3 weeks.
**3** Strain and pour into a glass bottle with a few sprigs of marjoram, a few marigold (calendula) flowers and a few cloves of peeled garlic.

## How to use

Take 1–1½ tablespoons in food daily.

## GROWING

Fill the bottom of a large square planter with drainage material and top up with a multipurpose compost. Place the artichoke in the centre, the golden marjoram in the front on one side and the purple basil on the other, once all danger of frosts has passed. Plant a marigold (calendula) either side of the back and the garlic where there is space. Water regularly and feed weekly.

### Plants you will need

+ 1 *Cynara scolymus* (globe artichoke)
+ 1 *Origanum majorana* (marjoram)
+ 2 *Ocimum basilicum* (basil)
+ 2 *Calendula officinalis* (marigold)
+ 3 *Allium sativum* (garlic)

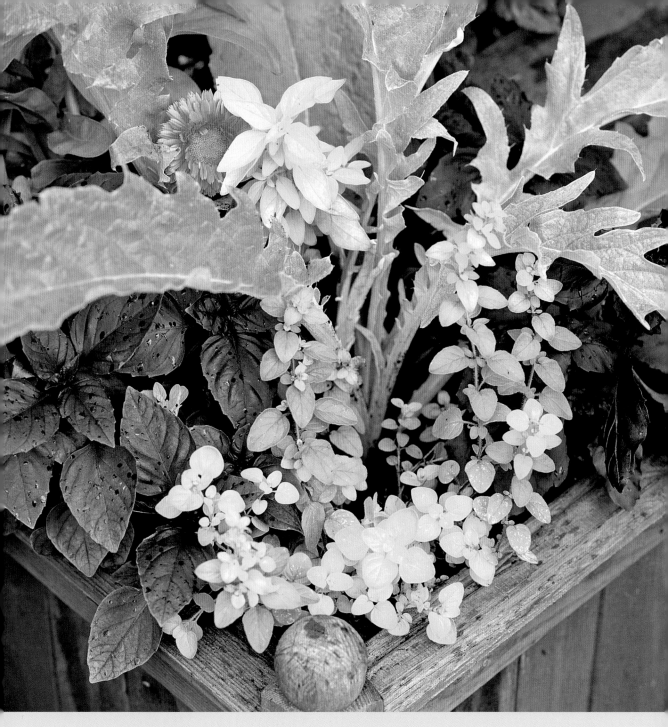

## You could also try...

Taking antioxidant herbs such as hawthorn, ginger and turmeric daily ◆ Eating antioxidant bilberries and elderberries. Oats also help lower cholesterol ◆ Eating plenty of fresh fruit and vegetables ◆ Taking supplements of shiitake and reishi mushrooms, garlic, B-complex supplement and fish oils ◆ Reducing high-fat foods, red meats, sugar, junk and fried foods ◆ Taking regular aerobic exercise.

# Toning compress

## For varicose veins

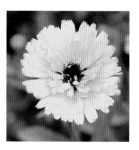

The magical combination of marigold (calendula), yarrow, agrimony and St John's wort helps tone swollen veins and relieve the aching that can accompany varicose veins. Yarrow is highly astringent, strengthens blood vessels, improves circulation and relieves pain and discomfort.

## Ingredients

⬧ 200 g (7 oz) each fresh or 100 g (3½ oz) dried yarrow, St John's wort and agrimony flowers and leaves, marigold (calendula) petals, chopped
⬧ 1 litre (1¾ pints) boiling water

**Makes 1 litre (1¾ pints) mixture**

## How to make

**1** Place the herb mixture in a teapot.
**2** Pour over boiling water. Leave to infuse for 30 minutes until it is lukewarm or cool.
**3** Strain and pour into a bowl.

## How to use

Soak a cloth in the infusion, wring it out gently and then apply to the area 2–3 times a day, or as often as you want.

**Hints and tips**
Avoid sitting or standing for long periods and be sure to take regular exercise.

## GROWING

Cover the bottom of a large pot with drainage material and top up with a multipurpose compost. Plant the St John's wort at the back, the agrimony on one side and the yarrow on the other. Place the marigolds (calendula) in the front. Deadhead the marigolds so that they continue to flower. Water regularly and feed weekly.

**Plants you will need**

⬧ 1 *Hypericum perforatum* (St John's wort)
⬧ 2 *Agrimonia eupatoria* (agrimony)
⬧ 1 *Achillea millefolium* (yarrow)
⬧ 2–3 *Calendula officinalis* (marigold)

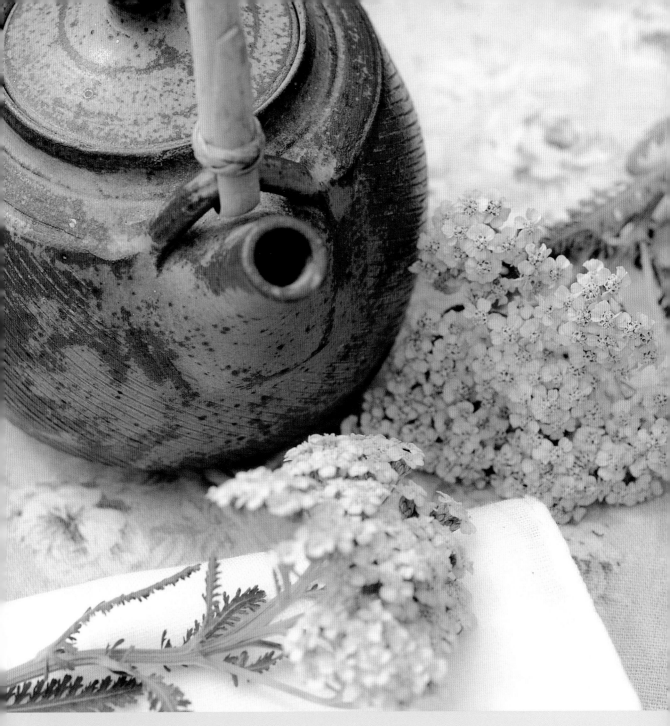

## You could also try...

Drinking teas of yarrow, limeflower or hawthorn to improve venous circulation ♦ Eating plenty of fruit and vegetables, especially bilberries and elderberries ♦ Taking supplements of zinc, vitamin E and vitamin C with bioflavonoids, garlic, gotu kola, ginkgo and horse chestnut ♦ Applying aloe vera gel or Manuka honey several times daily ♦ Using comfrey and calendula poultices alternated night and morning.

# Aromatic tisane

## For cystitis

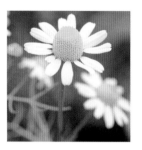

These herbs act as antiseptic diuretics, helping to combat infection and flush irritants from the urinary tract. Chamomile is soothing, relieving irritation and inflammation, while nasturtium, basil and parsley are antimicrobial and coriander relieves inflammation.

## Ingredients

- 100 g (3½ oz) each fresh or 50 g (2 oz) dried nasturtium, coriander, purple basil, parsley, chamomile
- 1 litre (1¾ pints) boiling water

**Makes 1 litre (1¾ pints) tisane**

## How to make

Place the herbs in a teapot. Pour over boiling water and leave to infuse for 10–15 minutes. Strain.

## How to use

Drink 1 cup every 1–2 hours for acute infections and 3 times a day as a preventative. Drink lukewarm to cool.

## GROWING

Line the hanging basket with moss or a similar permeable membrane to allow for drainage. Cover the lining with enough compost to reach the top of the basket. Plant the parsley and coriander in the centre of the basket. Place the chamomiles around them and the nasturtiums at the sides as they will more readily trail over the sides. Once all danger of frost has passed, plant the purple basil in the space at the front so that it can be seen. Water regularly and feed weekly.

**Plants you will need**

- 1 *Petroselinum crispum* (parsley)
- 4 *Coriandrum sativum* (coriander)
- 1 *Matricaria recutita* (German chamomile)
  *Anthemis nobilis/Chamaemelum nobile* (Roman chamomile)
- 2 *Tropaeolum majus* (nasturtium)
- 2 *Ocimum basilicum* (basil)

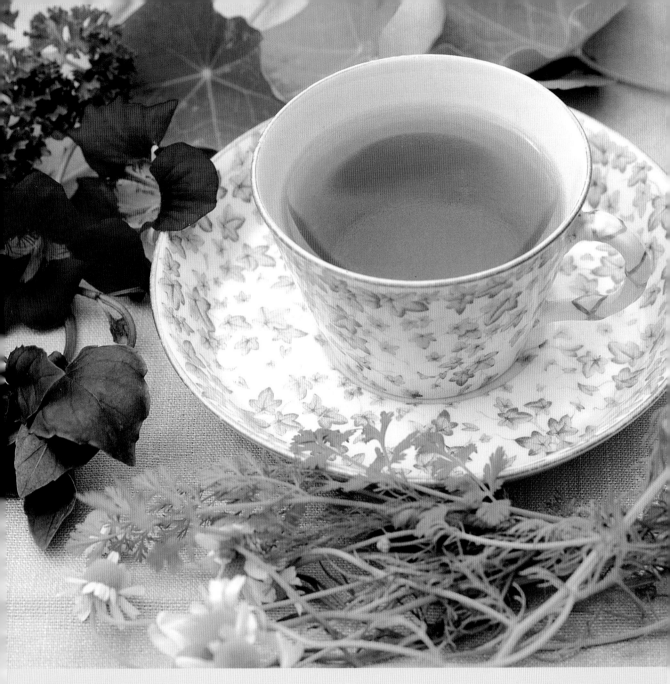

## You could also try...

Drinking lukewarm to cool teas of all or any of these
every hour or two in acute infections and 3 times
daily in chronic problems ♦ Drinking teas of uva ursi,
corn silk, chamomile, fennel, coriander, yarrow,
couch grass, marshmallow or horsetail frequently
♦ Sitting in a bath of strong chamomile tea for
10–15 minutes ♦ Drinking plenty of water or soothing
barley water through the day ♦ Eating soups and
juices made from carrots, parsley, asparagus, celery,
leeks and garlic ♦ Eating bilberries and drinking
cranberry juice to prevent bacteria from sticking to
the walls of the urinary tract.

# Strengthening salad
## For osteoporosis

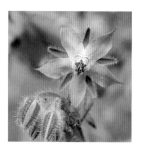

These herbs are rich in calcium, while rocket, nasturtiums dill, coriander and parsley also promote its digestion and absorption. Dandelion contains boron, calcium and magnesium, while dill, borage, coriander and calendula balance hormones and lessen risk of calcium loss.

## Ingredients

+ 150 g (5½ oz) mixture of lettuce and rocket
+ 5–10 leaves each dandelion, nasturtiums, borage, young plantain
+ 2 sprigs each dill, mint, coriander, parsley
+ 4 each marigold (calendula), borage, nasturtium flowers

Serves 2

## How to make

**1** Place the torn lettuce and rocket in the base of your salad bowl. Then put the dandelion, nasturtium, borage and plantain leaves in.
**2** Chop the dill, mint, coriander and parsley and then decorate with marigold (calendula), borage and nasturtium flowers.

## How to use

Serve with a simple dressing made with olive oil and balsamic vinegar.

**Did you know?**
Calcium, boron, magnesium, essential fatty acids and vitamin D are all vital for good bone density.

## GROWING

Using a tall planter with holes in the side, place drainage material in the bottom and fill with compost to the first level of holes. Plant the mint, rockets and nasturtiums through the holes, water and add more compost. Continue to plant through the holes staggering the mints, rockets and nasturtiums. Place the borage in the centre at the top, surround with marigold (calendula), nasturtium near the sides. Place the dill, parsley, plantain, rocket and coriander where they fit best. Water and feed.

**Plants you will need**

+ 1 *Mentha piperita* (peppermint)
+ 5 *Tropaeolum majus* (nasturtium)
+ 4 *Eruca vesicaria/sativa* (rocket)
+ 1 *Borago officinalis* (borage)
+ 3 *Calendula officinalis* (marigold)
+ 1 *Anethum graveolens* (dill)
+ 1 *Petroselinum crispum* (parsley)
+ 1 *Plantago major/minor/lanceolata* (plantain)
+ 1 *Coriandrum sativum* (coriander)

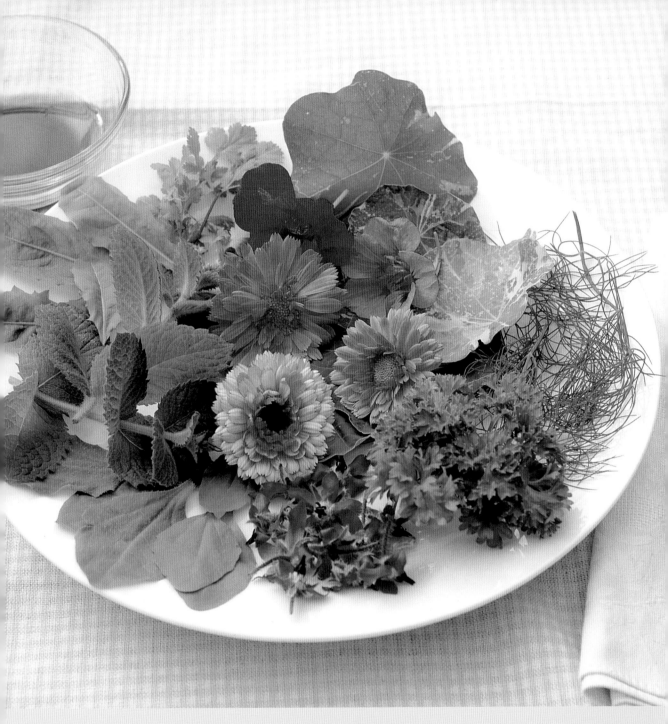

## You could also try...

Drinking teas of oestrogenic herbs, wild asparagus, Chinese angelica, red clover, calendula, wild yam, licorice, sage, hops or Siberian ginseng 3–4 times daily ◆ Adding herbs and spices to improve digestion and absorption to your diet including pepper, ginger, fennel, cumin or coriander ◆ Taking supplements of evening primrose or borage seed oil, vitamins E, D, magnesium and boron ◆ Taking plenty of exercise

# Waterfall juice

## For fluid retention

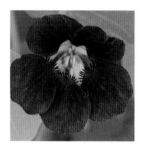

Fennel, coriander, dandelion, nasturtium and parsley, with their stimulating and penetrating tastes, make good adjuvants to the blander flavours of cucumber and celery. All aid the elimination of water through the kidneys and reduce fluid retention.

## Ingredients

- 75 g (3 oz) each wild celery leaves, dandelion leaves, fennel leaves and/or seeds, coriander leaves and/or seeds, nasturtium leaves and flowers and parsley leaves
- 1 bunch celery
- 1 cucumber

**Makes 350 ml (11 fl oz) juice**

## How to make

Put all the ingredients into an electric juicer.

## How to use

Drink 2 glasses of juice first thing in the morning for breakfast and also drink plenty of water throughout the day. Repeat over a few days for premenstrual fluid retention or over a few weeks if the problem is more chronic.

### Did you know...
Dandelion is particularly good as it is rich in potassium, iron, vitamins A and C. Its blood-cleansing property is especially valuable during a fast as it invigorates the body, improves digestive function and stimulates the liver and gallbladder.

## GROWING

Cover the bottom of a metal bucket with some drainage material and fill it with a multipurpose compost. Plant the wild celery and the parsley in the centre. Place the fennel on the right side, the dandelion on the left. Place the coriander on either side of the fennel and a single nasturtium next to each dandelion. Water and feed.

**Plants you will need**

- 2 *Apium graveolens* (wild celery)
- 1 *Petroselinum crispum* (parsley)
- 1 *Foeniculum vulgare* (fennel)
- 1 *Taraxacum officinale* (dandelion)
- 2 *Coriandrum sativum* (coriander)
- 2 *Tropaeolum majus* (nasturtium)

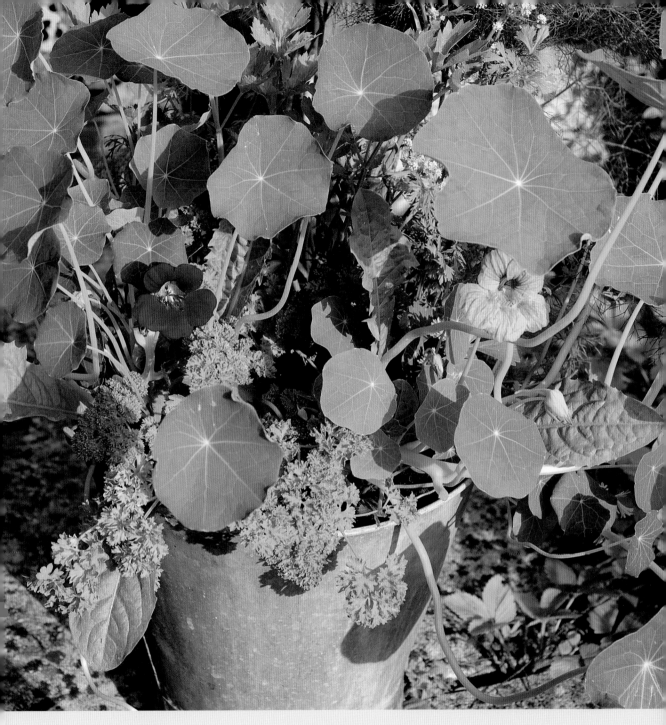

## You could also try...

Avoiding excess salt in your diet ♦ Eating plenty of potassium-containing foods such as bananas, tomatoes and green vegetables ♦ Drinking teas of diuretic herbs, celery seed, nettles, cleavers, fennel, coriander, meadowsweet, corn silk, chamomile and uva ursi 3–4 times daily ♦ Taking supplements of B complex ♦ Taking plenty of exercise ♦ Raising your feet when sitting • Avoiding tea, coffee and alcohol.

# Moon tea

## For menstrual problems

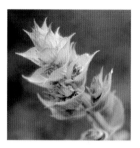

The combination of these aromatic herbs is designed to relieve symptoms due to hormonal fluctuations. These herbs help the liver break down hormones, regulate bleeding, benefit the nervous system and help relieve PMS, fluid retention, bloating and period pain.

## Ingredients

- 100 g (3½ oz) each fresh or 50 g (2 oz dried) rose, motherwort, lady's mantle, chamomile, clary sage
- 1 litre (1¾ pints) boiling water

Makes 1 litre (1¾ pints) tea

## How to make

Place the herbs in a teapot. Pour over boiling water and leave to infuse for 10–15 minutes. Strain.

**Hints and tips**
Rose relieves pain and spasm, stems heavy bleeding and relieves irritability and anxiety.

## How to use

Drink 1 cupful 3 times daily throughout the month. On the first day of your period, or whenever you experience most discomfort, drink throughout the day, as needed: up to 6 cups.

## GROWING

Cover the bottom of several matching pots with drainage material and fill with multipurpose compost. Plant a rose at the centre of the large pot and surround with chamomile. Plant the motherwort in another medium-sized pot, the clary sage in another and lady's mantle in the other. Water regularly and feed weekly.

**Plants you will need**

- 1 *Rosa spp* (rose)
- 3 *Matricaria recutita* (German chamomile) or *Anthemis nobilis/Chamaemelum nobile* (Roman chamomile)
- 1 *Leonurus cardiaca* (motherwort)
- 1 *Salvia sclarea* (clary sage)
- 1 *Alchemilla vulgaris* (lady's mantle)

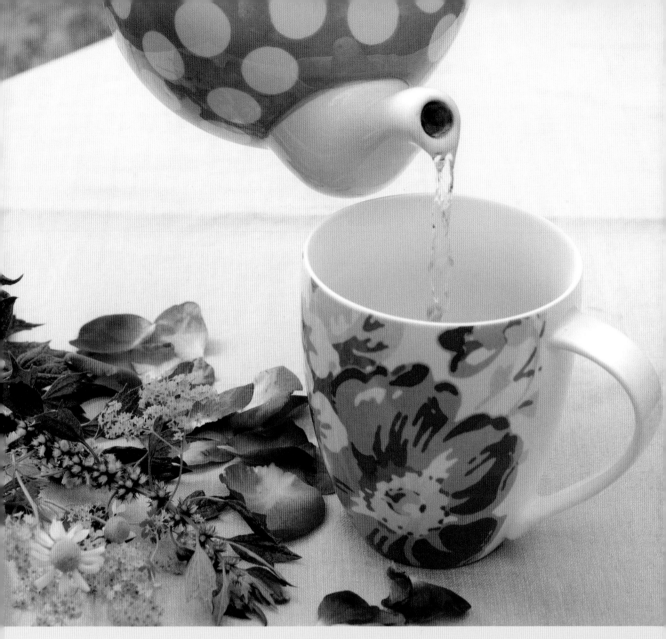

## You could also try...

Taking half a teaspoon of vitex agnus castus tincture half an hour before breakfast every day ♦ Drinking teas of licorice, burdock, wild asparagus and Chinese angelica 3 times daily to regulate hormones ♦ Drinking teas of motherwort, pasque flower or valerian every 2 hours, when necessary, to relieve period pain ♦ Drinking teas of yarrow, periwinkle or agrimony 3–6 times daily, as required, for heavy periods ♦ Eating iron-containing foods and herbs such as nettle, coriander leaf, kelp and dock to help combat anaemia ♦ Avoiding caffeine, alcohol, refined and junk foods ♦ Drinking teas of diuretic herbs, cleavers, dandelion or fennel to relieve fluid retention, bloating and breast discomfort ♦ Taking supplements of evening primrose oil, zinc, calcium, magnesium, vitamin E, and B complex.

# Balancing tincture

## For menopause symptoms

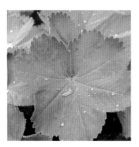

This blend supports hormonal and emotional balance. Motherwort, sage, rose and chamomile are cooling for hot flushes and are helpful to the liver. Sage promotes digestion and absorption, while rose and motherwort balance hormones and enhance mental equilibrium.

## Ingredients

- 250 g (9 oz) each fresh herbs or 100 g (3½ oz) dried red sage leaves, motherwort, lady's mantle, chamomile, rose petals
- 500 ml (17 fl oz) brandy or vodka

Makes 400 ml (14 fl oz) tincture

## How to make

**1** Place the herbs into a large glass jar.
**2** Pour over brandy or vodka and screw the lid on. Leave to macerate for a minimum of 2–3 weeks, up to 6 months.
**3** Press through a fine mesh sieve or use a wine press, squeezing as much of the liquid as possible before discarding the herb.
**4** Label clearly and store in dark glass bottles.

## How to use

Take 1–2 teaspoons 3 times daily in a little water. You may continue for at least 3 weeks, and up to 3 months, to benefit from the long-term benefits of the herbs.

## GROWING

Cover the bottom of a large square planter with drainage material and top up with multipurpose compost. Plant the rose in the centre at the back, put the motherwort on one side and the lady's mantle on the other. Plant the sage and chamomile at the front. Water regularly and feed weekly.

### Plants you will need

- 1 *Rosa spp* (rose)
- 1 *Leonurus cardiaca* (motherwort)
- 1 *Alchemilla vulgaris* (lady's mantle)
- 3 *Salvia officinalis* (sage)
- 2 *Matricaria recutita* (German chamomile) or *Anthemis nobilis/Chamaemelum nobile* (Roman chamomile)

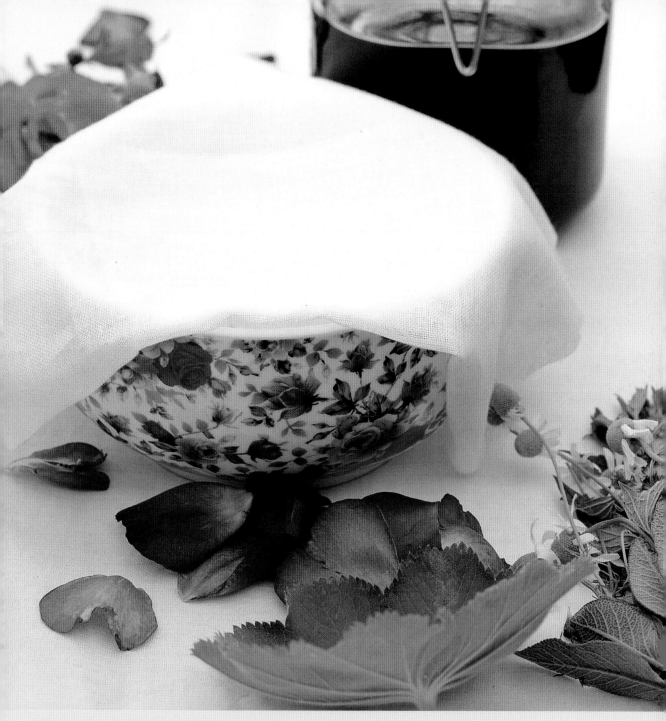

## You could also try...

Drinking teas of wild asparagus, red clover, wild yam, Chinese angelica, Siberian ginseng, licorice or black cohosh to balance hormones 3–4 times daily ♦ Drinking teas of chamomile, hops, vervain, wild oats and lemon balm 3–6 times daily for anxiety and insomnia with night sweats ♦ Taking supplements of borage seed or evening primrose oil, vitamin E, calcium and magnesium.

# Healing oil

## For cuts and wounds

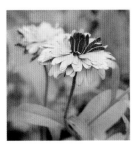

Herbs can provide instant first aid for grazes, cuts and wounds. Plantain and yarrow stop bleeding and soothe pain, while marigold (calendula) and lavender flowers reduce inflammation, prevent infection and promote healing. A base of virgin coconut oil can speed healing.

## Ingredients

- 150 g (5½ oz) each yarrow leaves and flowers, marigold (calendula) petals, lavender flowers, plantain leaves
- 250 ml (9 fl oz) virgin coconut oil, warmed

**Makes 250 ml (9 fl oz) oil**

## How to make

**1** Wash and pat dry enough fresh herbs to fill your chosen clean glass jar.

**2** Pour over warmed coconut oil (it becomes solid at low temperatures) until it covers the herbs and screw the lid on as tight as possible.

**3** Place the jar in the sun for 3 weeks, shaking it now and again.

**4** Strain the oil through a fine mesh sieve or clean muslin cloth into bottles, which need to be stored in a cool place.

## How to use

Apply 3–6 times daily or as required.

### Hints and tips

Marigold (calendula) flowers hold pride of place as a first-aid remedy. They stem bleeding, speed healing and prevent infection.

## GROWING

Cover the bottom of a large square pot with drainage material and fill with a multipurpose compost. Plant the lavender at the centre, the marigolds (calendula) around the lavender, the plantain in one corner, yarrow in another. Water regularly and feed weekly.

### Plants you will need

- 1 *Lavandula officinalis* (lavender)
- 5 *Calendula officinalis* (marigold)
- 1 *Plantago major/minor/lanceolata* (plantain)
- 1 *Achillea millefolium* (yarrow)

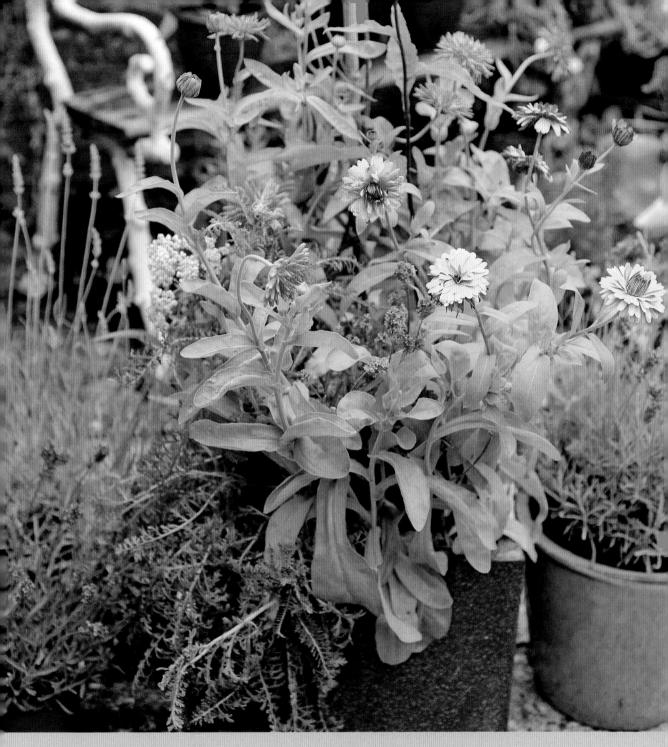

## You could also try...

Applying freshly crushed leaves of plantain, yarrow, comfrey or agrimony to stop bleeding ♦ Applying tinctures of yarrow, calendula, plantain, comfrey or agrimony directly to gauze and putting it over the wound ♦ Bathing the area with infusions of lavender and calendula ♦ Covering with calendula cream.

# Soothing compress

## For minor burns and scalds

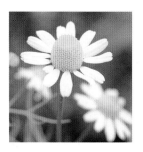

If your scald or burn is small, you can treat it at home by using this healing compress. Aloe vera gel is renowned for its soothing effect and its ability to heal quickly. Lavender and marigold (calendula) are healers with antiseptic properties, while plantain and coriander ease pain and burning.

## Ingredients

- 60 g (2½ oz) each fresh or 30 g (1 oz) dried marigold (calendula) petals, plantain and coriander leaves, lavender flowers
- 500 ml (17 fl oz) boiling water
- 20 ml (1 fl oz) aloe vera gel

**Makes 500 ml (17 fl oz) liquid**

## How to make

**1** Immerse the burnt area in cold water for 5–10 minutes or until pain subsides.
**2** Place the mixture of herbs in a teapot and pour over the boiling water.
**3** Infuse for 10–15 minutes and allow to cool.
**4** Mix in the aloe vera gel.

## How to use

Soak a clean cloth in the mixture, wring it out and apply gently to the area, repeating until the pain subsides. Apply neat aloe vera gel while waiting for the tea to cool if there is much pain. Do not burst any blisters that form.

## GROWING

Cover the bottom of a wooden planter with drainage material and fill with multipurpose compost. Place the lavender at the back, the marigolds (calendula) in the corners, the aloe vera on one side, the plantain on the other and the chamomiles in the spaces in between. Water and feed.

**Plants you will need**

- 1 *Lavandula officinalis* (lavender)
- 3 *Calendula officinalis* (marigold)
- 1 *Aloe barbadensis* (aloe vera)
- 1 *Plantago major/minor/lanceolata* (plantain)
- 3 *Matricaria recutita* (German chamomile) or *Anthemis nobilis/Chamaemelum nobile* (Roman chamomile)

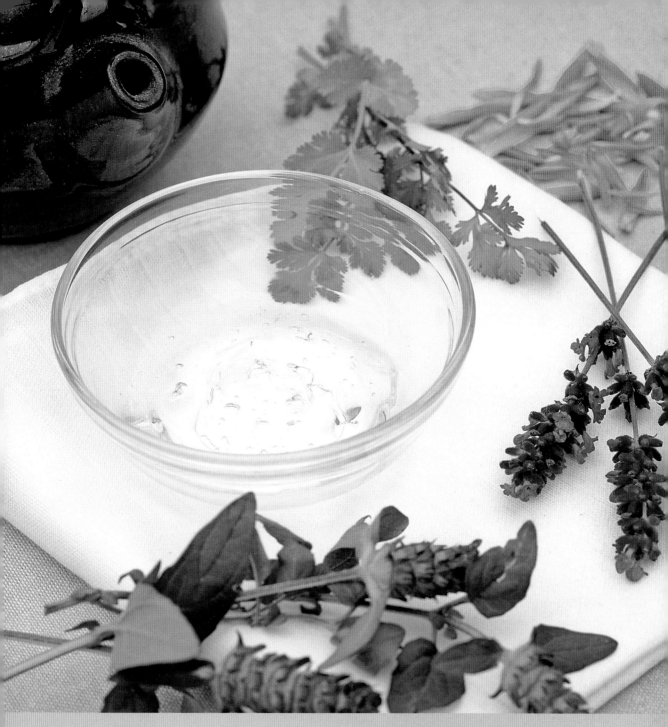

## You could also try...

Raising the affected area slightly to slow blood flow to the area and ease the pain ♦ Applying neat lavender oil ♦ Applying a poultice made with the herbs (see left) or using comfrey leaves ♦ Alternating neat lavender oil with comfrey ointment repeatedly, until the pain subsides ♦ Covering the area loosely with a clean, dry dressing; if it sticks to the skin soak it off with warm infusion of calendula.

# Herbal sting rubs

## For bites and stings

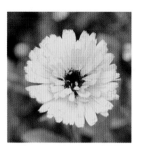

Rubbing herbs directly on bites and stings can bring instant relief. Lavender and basil help prevent swelling and relieve pain. Crushed plantain leaves draw out toxins and lavender flowers are healing and anti-inflammatory; both are excellent for wasp stings and mosquito bites.

## Ingredients

♦ Any of the following:
1 marigold (calendula) flower,
1–2 lavender flowers, 1–2
basil leaves, 1 leaf aloe vera,
1 leaf plantain

## How to make

Using the fresh herb, rub it between your fingers and then rub it on to the site of the bite or sting.

### Warning
Seek IMMEDIATE medical attention if your tongue swells, you have difficulty breathing or a sudden rash after being stung by a bee.

## How to use

First extract the sting, if you are stung by a bee, then rub the fresh herbs on to the sting for a few minutes. Repeat several times if necessary. When using aloe vera use the gel inside the leaf.

## GROWING

Cover the bottom of two medium-sized pots with drainage material and top up with multipurpose compost. Plant the lavender and plantain in the centre of one pot and the marigolds (calendula) on either side. In the other pot put a lemon basil at the centre with aloe vera at either side once all danger of frost has passed. Water regularly and feed weekly.

### Plants you will need

♦ 1 *Plantago major/minor/lanceolata* (plantain)
♦ 2 *Calendula officinalis* (marigold)
♦ 1 *Lavandula officinalis* (lavender)
♦ 1 *Ocimum basilicum* (lemon basil)
♦ 4 small *Aloe barbadensis* (aloe vera)

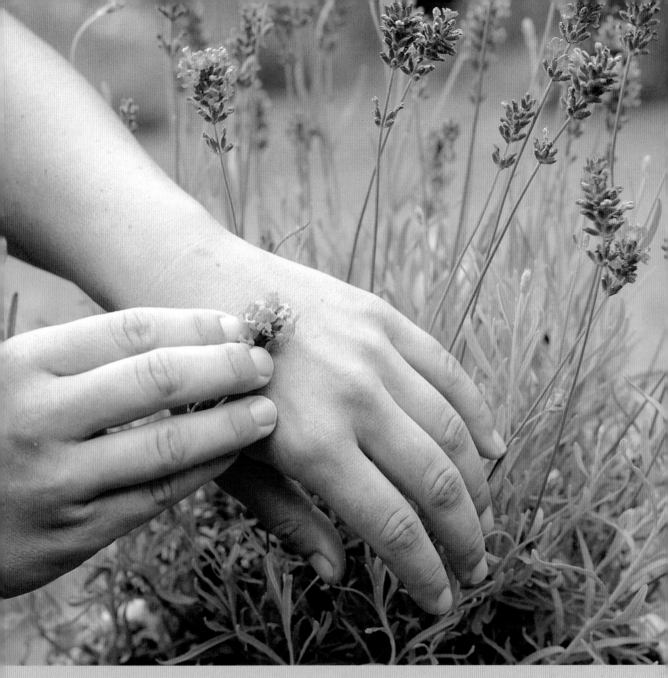

## You could also try...

Chewing plantain leaves, mixing them well with your saliva and then applying them to stings • Applying raw garlic to ant stings ✦ Applying witch hazel, lemon juice or cider vinegar to mosquito bites ✦ Using insect-repellent oil made from 5 drops of citronella, tea tree, lavender or rosemary oil in 1 teaspoon of sesame oil ✦ Applying a few drops of lavender essential oil ✦ Applying distilled witch hazel, infusion of sage, bicarbonate of soda or sliced lemon to bee stings ✦ Infusing thyme and rosemary in apple cider vinegar and dabbing the vinegar on bites to draw out any poison and prevent swelling.

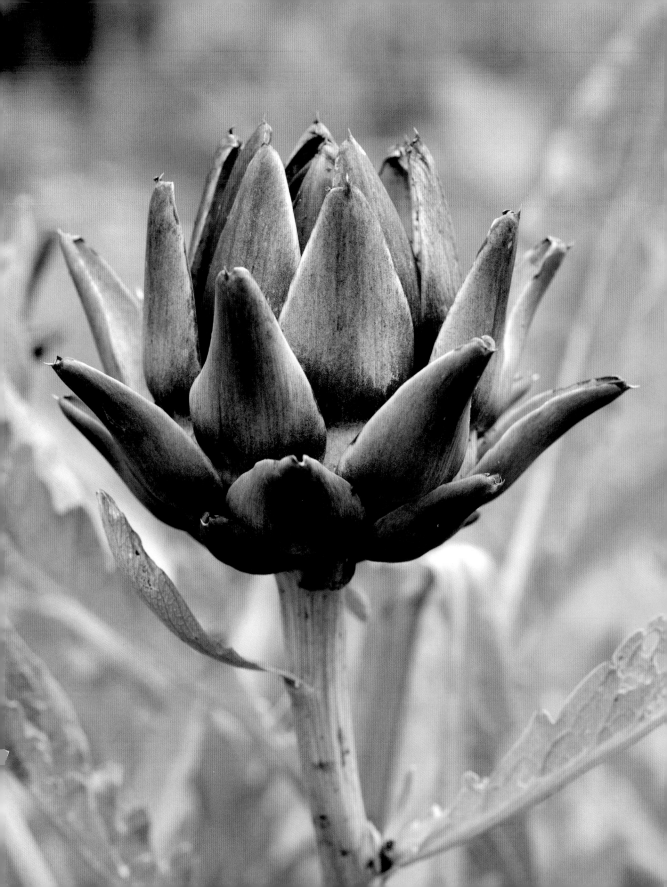

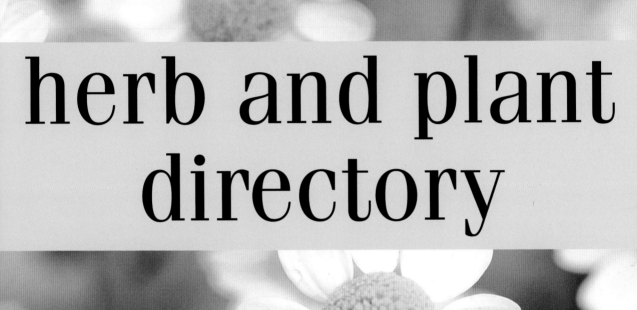

# herb and plant directory

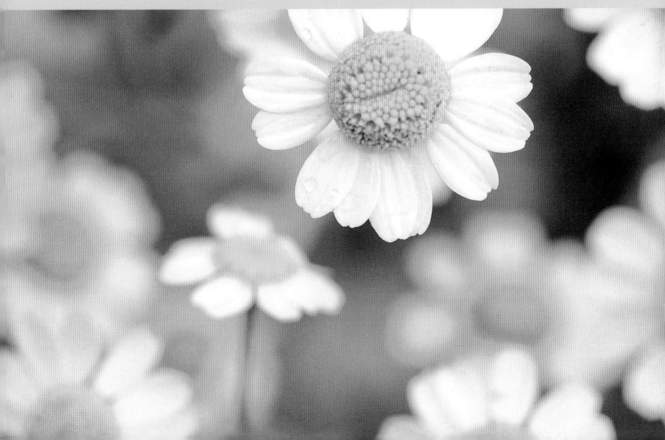

# Achillea millefolium
## Yarrow

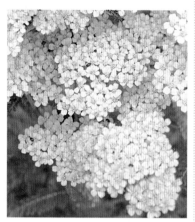

Yarrow has aromatic leaves and it grows in hedgerows, lanes and meadows. It has white or pink flowers and is quite drought-resistant. The leaves and flowers make an excellent remedy, with their antiseptic, anti-inflammatory and astringent actions and silica to promote tissue repair. Yarrow speeds healing of wounds, ulcers, burns and in creams it can be applied to varicose veins, haemorrhoids and skin conditions.

A tea or tincture makes a good remedy for diarrhoea, wind, indigestion and inflammatory problems. It stimulates the appetite, enhances digestion and absorption and relaxes gut tension. It helps regulate the menstrual cycle and supports the nervous system. In a hot tea it increases sweating and is a good remedy for fevers, colds, flu and catarrh. It is an excellent circulatory remedy, helping to lower blood pressure and relieve poor circulation.

# Agrimonia eupatoria
## Agrimony

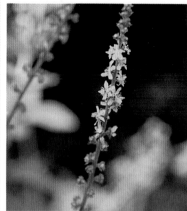

Agrimony is a pretty, hardy perennial with slender, long spikes of apricot-scented, pale-yellow flowers, often found growing wild in summer hedgerows, meadows and waste ground.

The leaves and flowers make a great remedy for improving your digestion and absorption of food and supporting the liver in its detoxifying work. Their astringent tannins protect the gut lining from irritation and inflammation and help to heal inflammatory problems such as gastritis, colitis and peptic ulcers. You can use agrimony to relieve diarrhoea and to treat liver and gall-bladder problems. Its diuretic effects help cleanse toxins from the system, which is helpful in arthritis and gout. Agrimony makes a good gargle for sore throats and eyewash for inflamed eyes.

# Alchemilla vulgaris
## Lady's mantle

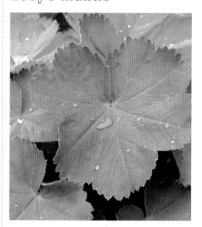

Lady's mantle is an attractive hardy perennial with distinctive pale-green leaves and tiny, lacy yellow-green flowers. This plant is an excellent astringent and anti-inflammatory for women; the leaves and flowers are used for heavy, painful or irregular periods, for prolonged bleeding due to fibroids or when peri-menopausal, to aid contractions and to enhance recovery. Lady's mantle is helpful in genito-urinary infections, fibroids and pelvic inflammatory disease.

It is also good for the digestive tract, relieving diarrhoea and inflammatory problems such as gastritis, colitis or gastro-enteritis and for the urinary system as it has diuretic properties. An infusion or dilute tincture makes an excellent douche for vaginal infections, a skin lotion for rashes, cuts and abrasions and a gargle for sore throats.

**Caution:** Avoid during pregnancy.

# Allium sativum
## Garlic

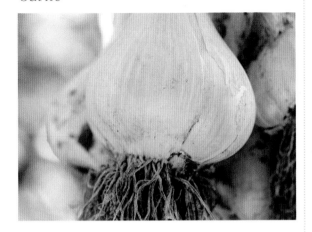

This powerful-smelling perennial makes an excellent companion plant, especially under roses, to keep aphids away. Garlic is an excellent remedy for infections, having antibacterial, antiviral, antiparasitic and antifungal properties. It exerts its effects throughout the digestive, respiratory and urinary systems, disinfecting as it goes, enhancing immunity and remedying coughs, colds, stomach and bowel infections, and cystitis.

It also acts as a decongestant, is good for catarrh and hay fever, and as an expectorant – useful when treating coughs and asthma. Garlic is a wonderful medicine for the heart and circulation, lowering raised blood pressure and harmful cholesterol levels. It reduces the tendency to blood clotting, thereby helping to reduce heart attacks and strokes. The antioxidants help to guard against degenerative disease, heart disease and cancer. In addition the sulphur compounds contained in garlic have anti-tumour properties. Garlic also helps the body withstand the ageing process and at the same time garlic acts as an invigorating tonic – a veritable 'elixir of life'.

**Caution:** Garlic needs to be eaten raw to benefit most from its therapeutic action. Cooking destroys around 95 per cent of its medicinal value. Garlic capsules may be effective.

# Aloe barbadensis
## Aloe vera

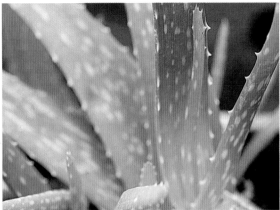

A succulent plant, indigenous to eastern and southern Africa, found growing happily in most tropical places. This could include sunny window ledges in your home as it prefers to grow indoors in temperate climates. The clear mucilaginous gel inside the juicy leaves is wonderful for soothing and healing the skin. You can use it for minor burns, sunburn, after radiation therapy, wounds, cuts and abrasions, haemorrhoids, and sensitive and allergic skin conditions such as acne, eczema and psoriasis. It also rejuvenates the skin and may reduce wrinkles.

When it is mixed with water it is known as aloe juice and is used for its cooling and moistening effect for problems associated with excess heat and inflammation. It is a wonderful aid for digestion, increasing secretion of digestive enzymes, balancing stomach acid; soothing and protecting your gut lining. You can use it for treating colitis, peptic ulcers, irritable bowel syndrome and inflammatory bowel disease. It is a mild laxative, clearing toxins and heat from the bowel and combating infection. It also regulates sugar and fat metabolism; helpful in diabetes and if you want to lose weight. Aloe enhances immunity and is antiviral, antifungal, antibacterial and can be used as a probiotic. It is anti-inflammatory and detoxifying for arthritis, great for PMS and can reduce hot flushes during menopause.

# Althaea officinalis
## Marshmallow

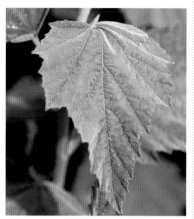

Marshmallow is a lovely stately perennial with soft velvety leaves and soft-pink flowers, often found growing in marshes by the sea. Butterflies love it.

Marshmallow is the most soothing of medicines. The leaves, flowers and root are wonderful for internal and external irritation and inflammation. It is antimicrobial and immune-enhancing, stimulating production of white blood cells and aiding the body's fight against infection. A mild expectorant, marshmallow soothes dry coughs, sore throats, asthma, croup and bronchitis. It eases digestive problems and is a soothing diuretic, relieving cystitis and an irritable bladder. Marshmallow leaves can be rubbed on bites and stings, scalds and burns, sunburn and skin rashes. A warm poultice will help draw out splinters, while a gargle can be used for sore throats and inflamed gums.

# Ancthum gravcolcns
## Dill

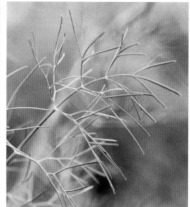

Dill, originally from the Mediterranean, where it is often found wild, is a highly aromatic annual with feathery leaves and umbels of tiny yellow flowers. The leaves, with their delicious aniseed taste, are used in salads, vegetable, meat and fish dishes, while the seeds are used as a pickling spice.

The mildly pungent taste of dill stimulates the flow of digestive juices, whetting the appetite and enhancing digestion and absorption. Its muscle-relaxing effect releases tension and ensures the proper movement of food and wastes along the gut. Decoctions of the seeds can help relieve colic and wind, indigestion and nausea, constipation and diarrhoea. Dill's relaxant effect can soothe irritating coughs and asthma. In the reproductive tract dill helps relieve period pain and regulate menstruation – long used as a remedy to ease childbirth and stimulate milk production.

# Apium graveolens
## Wild celery

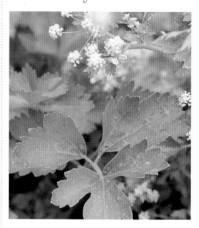

Wild celery is a tall, aromatic biennial with a fleshy, bulbous root and is the original celery from which we cultivated the familiar vegetable. It can be found growing wild in damp and marshy ground.

All parts of wild celery can be used as food and medicine. It has a similar action to parsley and they both contain apiol, an antiseptic constituent with an affinity for the urinary system. It has a diuretic effect, good for fluid retention and cystitis and helps clear toxins from the system. The leaves and the seed make an excellent remedy for arthritis and gout, as well as a tonic to the digestive tract, and have an uplifting effect upon the nervous system.

# Borago officinalis
## Borage

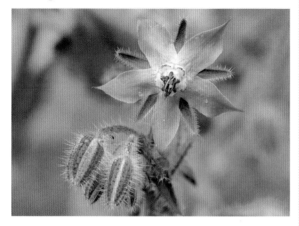

# Calendula officinalis
## Marigold

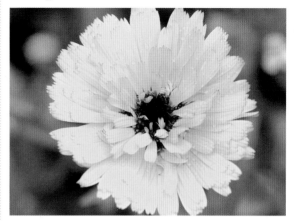

Borage is a lovely annual with pretty bright-blue, star-shaped flowers, loved by bees. The young leaves are highly nutritious, imparting their cucumber taste to salads, while the flowers can brighten summer drinks and puddings. When it is grown near tomatoes, it deters pests.

You can use borage leaves and flowers to relieve tension and anxiety and to lift the spirits. Their affinity for the adrenal glands helps to support the body during times of stress.

Borage has a cooling and cleansing effect, clearing heat and toxins from the body by increasing perspiration and urination. It can be used in recipes for arthritis, skin problems, fevers and childhood infections such as measles and chicken pox.

With its decongestant and soothing, expectorant effect, borage is good when treating colds, catarrh, coughs and chest infections. It also increases milk flow during breastfeeding. The seeds contain gamma linoleic acid (GLA), which is excellent for helping hormonal problems, allergies and arthritis.

Marigold (calendula) flowers have astringent and antiseptic properties and help fight off infections, including colds and flu, herpes virus, pelvic and bowel infections including enteritis, amoebae and worms, and fungal infections. In the digestive tract, marigolds relieve irritation and promote healing of the gastric and bowel lining, relieving gastritis, peptic ulcers, colitis and diverticulitis. The bitters stimulate the appetite, enhance digestion and absorption and improve liver and gall-bladder function. Hot marigold tea increases circulation and promotes sweating, helping to relieve fevers, improve blood and lymphatic circulation and enable the body to throw off toxins. Its diuretic action aids elimination of fluid and toxins. Marigolds have an affinity to the female reproductive system and help menstruation and period problems, endometriosis and cysts. Their hormonal properties help relieve symptoms such as hot flushes.

Marigolds help stop bleeding and speed healing of cuts and grazes, and their astringent, antiseptic properties are excellent for healing sores and ulcers, varicose veins and haemorrhoids, minor burns and scalds, chilblains and cold sores, slow-healing wounds and infections, as well as for treating skin problems such as eczema.

**Caution:** Avoid during pregnancy.

# Capsicum frutescens
## Cayenne pepper

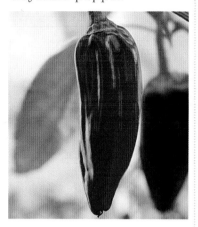

Chilli peppers are rich in beta-carotene and vitamin C, natural antioxidants that protect against degenerative disease, cancer, and cardiovascular disease such as atherosclerosis and angina.

Eating chillis regularly enhances immunity and helps fight off infections and allergies. They bring down fevers, clear catarrh and overcome infection. Chillis stimulate digestion, improving appetite and absorption. In the reproductive system, their warming properties have a muscle-relaxing effect, relieving pain caused by poor circulation and bringing on delayed periods. They help prevent blood clots and can lower harmful cholesterol by reducing the liver's production of cholesterol and triglycerides. Chilli peppers are often used as stimulants in ointments and liniments to relieve arthritic and muscular pain, neuralgia, bruises, back pain and unbroken chilblains.

# Carum carvi
## Caraway

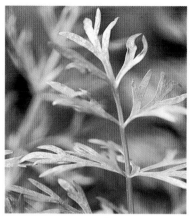

An attractive biennial and member of the carrot family, caraway has bright-green, feathery leaves and umbels of white flowers in summer.

The parsley-like smell of the leaves and the spicy taste of the seeds are imparted by an aromatic, volatile oil that stimulates digestion while relaxing the muscles in the digestive tract. It improves appetite, digestion and absorption by increasing the flow of digestive juices. Caraway seeds have a warming effect by increasing blood flow throughout the body. You can use them for symptoms associated with cold, including tiredness, lethargy, weak digestion and lowered immunity. They have an invigorating and uplifting effect and their antiseptic, volatile oils help the body's fight against infection. A hot decoction makes a good expectorant and decongestant for bronchial catarrh and chest infections. Gargling with it will help soothe a sore throat and laryngitis.

# Centella/Hydrocotyle
## asiatica Gotu kola

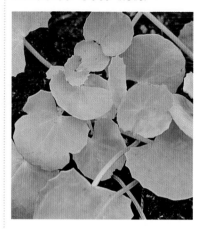

Gotu kola is renowned for its ability to enhance memory and concentration. A brain tonic, the leaves can boost brain power, help children with autism and learning difficulties. It can help protect against ageing and Alzheimer's. Gotu kola is a great remedy for relieving stress, anxiety, insomnia and depression. Its anticonvulsant actions can help epilepsy. It has a calming effect in the digestive system. Its antibacterial action may contribute to its anti-ulcer properties.

Gotu kola has an ability to speed the healing of wounds and scars by increasing the circulation to the area. It can help resolve inflammatory skin problems, oedema, cellulite, poor venous circulation and varicose veins. It is particularly recommended for post-operative use, and in addition it prevents bleeding and helps in anaemia. It also clears toxins, allays inflammation.

# Chelidonium majus
## Greater celandine

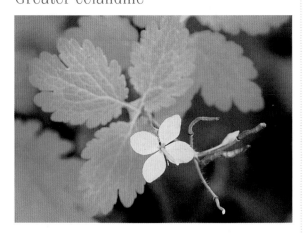

# Chrysanthemum parthenium/
## Tanacetum parthenium Feverfew

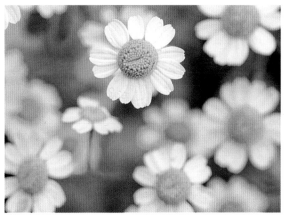

The greater celandine is an attractive perennial, closely related to the horned poppy, found growing wild on waste ground, in cultivated earth, against walls and in small cracks in walls and pavements. All parts of the plant contain a bitter and acrid-tasting bright-orange latex.

Traditionally greater celandine leaves and flowers are used for inflammatory and infectious eye problems and professional herbalists prescribe it for infections of the liver and gall bladder and for gall stones. It has a cleansing action through diuretic effect on the liver, the great detoxifying organ of the body. It makes a good remedy for arthritis, gout, allergies and skin problems and due to its narcotic properties, for insomnia and stress-related problems. The fresh-orange latex makes an excellent paint for getting rid of warts.

**Caution:** Internal use is not recommended.

Feverfew is an attractive hardy perennial with aromatic lacy-edged leaves and daisy flowers that are loved by bees. It is excellent in the herb garden as its cheerful flowers bloom in late summer, when many others have gone over.

Feverfew is famous as a remedy for headaches and migraine; as a preventative the fresh leaves can be eaten with other food, perhaps in a salad, or with crackers, every day. The bitter taste enhances digestion and liver function and thereby helps to clear toxins and heat from the body.

Feverfew can also be used as an anti-inflammatory for arthritis, and to relieve nerve pain such as shingles and sciatica. Taken in a hot infusion, it reduces fevers and acts as a decongestant for colds and catarrh. It relieves allergies such as hayfever and asthma, due to its antihistamine action,

**Caution:** Avoid taking in pregnancy. Fresh leaves eaten alone may cause mouth ulcers.

# Coriandrum sativum
## Coriander

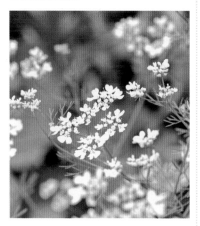

Coriander's tasty seeds are great for digestion, enhancing appetite and improving digestion and absorption of nutrients and preventing bloating. Coriander calms nerves and relaxes tense muscles and so is useful for relieving stress-related digestive disorders as well as period pain and childbirth contractions. The leaves and seeds have a cooling, cleansing effect, helping bring down fevers. It is helpful in inflammatory problems, including cystitis, conjunctivitis, sore throats, arthritis and skin rashes. The juice of the leaves helps clear toxins and is useful in allergies. A cold decoction of the seeds can help menopausal flushes and night sweats. Taken regularly coriander has an energizing effect. A hot decoction of the seeds makes a good remedy for fevers, colds, flu, catarrh and bronchial congestion, and can be used as a gargle for sore throats. The volatile oils in the seeds have antibacterial properties.

# Cynara scolymus
## Globe artichoke

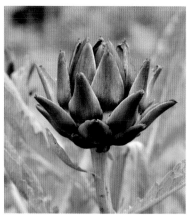

Globe artichoke is an impressive hardy perennial, ornamental as well as edible, with its silvery leaves and large grey-blue, thistle-like flowers. The flower heads are popular as a vegetable, especially in Mediterranean countries.

Artichoke leaves have the ability to lower cholesterol and to protect the heart and arteries from degenerative disease. The leaves can be used to improve liver and gall-bladder function and are used for poor appetite and digestion, heartburn, nausea and skin problems such as acne, eczema and urticaria. Their diuretic properties enhance the elimination of fluid and toxins from the system. So with its beneficial action on the liver, as well as on the kidneys, artichoke makes a good cleansing remedy, helping to clear toxins and to relieve arthritis and gout.

# Echinacea angustifolia
## Purple coneflower

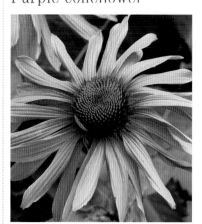

Purple coneflower is a perennial plant with striking pink-purple, daisy-like flowers. All parts of the plant, but particularly the root, are renowned for their ability to boost immunity and make an excellent remedy for fevers and all kinds of infections, acute or chronic. It has antibacterial, antiviral and anti-fungal actions, as well as anti-allergenic properties. Its anti-inflammatory properties are excellent for relieving arthritis and gout, skin disease and problems such as pelvic inflammatory disease. The tincture makes a good mouthwash for gum disease and a wash for wounds, sores and stings.

For best effect echinacea should be taken at the first signs of acute infection every two hours, and as a preventative or for chronic infections it can be taken three times daily for up to three weeks at a time.

# Eruca vesicaria/sativa
## Rocket

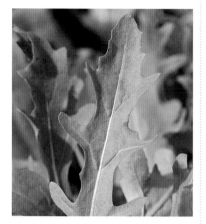

Rocket, with its popular fiery salad leaves grows wild in many parts of Europe and Asia. The leaves are rich in vitamins A and C and minerals, notably iron, calcium and potassium. Rocket was once eaten to prevent scurvy, and given as an emetic to induce vomiting to clear toxins from the stomach. Rocket leaves are best picked young to add to salads and go better with bland-tasting salad vegetables. When used medicinally they are usually picked later, when their pungency is more obvious.

The stimulating properties of rocket leaves can be felt in the digestive tract, where they enhance digestion and absorption and in the respiratory tract, where they clear congestion by loosening phlegm and relieve coughs, colds, catarrh and bronchial congestion. The natural antioxidants in the leaves enhance immunity and prevent damage caused by free radicals.

# Eschscholzia californica
## California poppy

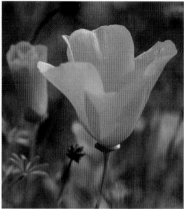

This vibrant yellow-orange flower is a safe sedative for adults and children alike and has a reputation as a non-addictive alternative to the opium poppy.

Taken as a tea or tincture, all parts of the plant, including the roots and seed pots, can calm agitation, anxiety, tension and insomnia. Its pain-killing and relaxing effects can help relieve migraine, headaches, neuralgia, back and muscle pain, arthritis, sciatica and shingles. You can even apply it to areas of pain such as toothache and headaches. It helps to balance emotions, reduces stress and is particularly helpful in withdrawal from addiction to alcohol, drugs or tobacco. By calming the nervous system, California poppy influences the heart and circulation; it slows a rapid heart, relieves palpitations, and reduces blood pressure. Its wonderful muscle-relaxing effects help relieve colic in the stomach, bowel and gall bladder.

# Eupatorium perfoliatum Boneset

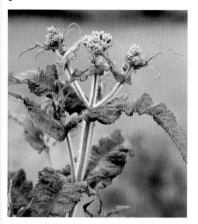

Native to eastern North America, where it is found growing in meadows and marshland, boneset was renowned among native Americans, who used it for flu and fevers. In fact, the plant was so named because it can relieve that aching feeling that comes with flu that feels as if it penetrates to the very bones.

The leaves and flowers boost immunity, combating bacterial and viral infections, including herpes, colds and flu. A hot tea can help you sweat out a fever and clear heat and toxins. It can also relieve catarrhal congestion that comes with hay fever, bronchitis, colds and coughs. When cool the tea can be used as a body wash to bring down fevers. Through its cleansing action on the liver and laxative effect it clears toxins from the digestive tract and this is useful in arthritis, skin conditions and worms.

# Filipendula ulmaria
## Meadowsweet

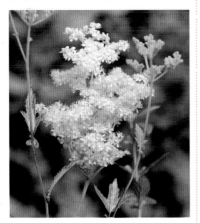

The leaves and flowers of meadowsweet make an excellent remedy for a range of digestive disorders, including acidity, gastritis and ulcers. A tea or tincture will relieve wind, diarrhoea, IBS, enteritis and colic, flatulence and distension and has an antiseptic as well as anti-inflammatory action.

Meadowsweet is rich in vitamin C, iron, calcium, magnesium and silica and speeds healing of connective tissue.Its anti-inflammatory effect relieves pain and swelling in arthritis and gout, its diuretic action helps eliminate excess fluid and toxins from the body, while its analgesic action soothes pain, not only joint pain but also headaches and neuralgia. A hot tea helps reduce fevers and to bring out rashes in eruptive infections and speed recovery. It has a reputation for softening deposits in the body and cholesterol build up in the arteries.

# Foeniculum vulgare
## Fennel

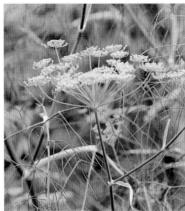

Fennel is an attractive, statuesque perennial with blue-green feathery leaves and large umbels of flowers, followed by tasty aromatic seeds.

Fennel has a warming and relaxing effect throughout the digestive tract, increasing appetite, digestion and absorption, particularly of carbohydrates and fats. It helps to relieve tension and spasm causing colic in the gut. Drinking fennel tea settles the stomach and relieves wind, nausea, indigestion and heartburn. As a diuretic, fennel increases elimination of fluid and toxins and is well known as a remedy for fluid retention and as a cleansing remedy for arthritis and cellulite. Its muscle-relaxing effects extend to the uterus, where it can help reduce period pains, while its hormone-like action is used to regulate the menstrual cycle and is helpful during the menopause. In the respiratory system fennel helps loosen tight coughs and clear congestion.

# Fragaria vesca
## Wild strawberry

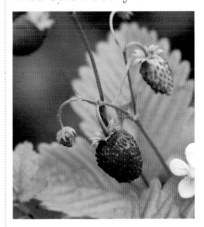

Strawberry leaves have astringent properties and can be used as gargles and mouthwashes. The roots have bitter properties and stimulate the liver and enhance digestion. The fruits are high in vitamin C and have been used to relieve fevers, for fluid retention, constipation and gout. They are highly nutritious, rich in vitamins and minerals.

The calcium and magnesium in the fruit and the leaves help support the nervous system, lifting the spirits and calming the nerves. The seeds are rich in pectin, providing a mild laxative effect and helping to reduce harmful cholesterol levels. Strawberries are good for preventing heart and arterial disease, heart attacks and strokes. However, the seeds may cause irritation to those with inflammatory digestive problems.

**Caution:** Excessive consumption can lead to allergic reactions.

## Glechoma/Nepeta hederacea Ground ivy

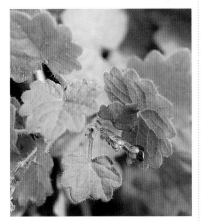

Ground ivy is a pleasant-tasting remedy, valued for its mild antiseptic and expectorant properties, useful for colds, flu, coughs and chest infections. As a gentle herb, it is perfect for children with catarrhal problems of the ear, nose and throat, congestive headaches and bronchial phlegm and helps to relieve fevers when taken as a hot tea.

It enhances the appetite, digestion and absorption of nutrients and protects the lining of the gut from irritation and inflammation. It can be used for indigestion, wind, bloating, nausea and diarrhoea and was traditionally used for expelling worms. Its diuretic action helps fluid retention, clears toxins from the system and is helpful in cystitis and urinary tract infections. The tea or dilute tincture can be used as a gargle for sore throats and a lotion to bathe inflamed eyes and heal cuts and abrasions.

## Hypericum perforatum St John's wort

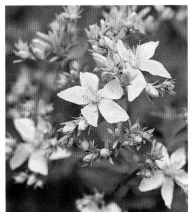

St John's wort has an affinity for the nervous system, easing tension and anxiety and is famous for lifting depression. It increases sensitivity to sunlight and is recommended for seasonal affective disorder (SAD) and jet lag. It is excellent for emotional problems during the menopause and is one of the best herbs for relieving pain.

In the digestive tract it is a good astringent and antimicrobial remedy for gastroenteritis, diarrhoea and dysentery, and can speed healing of peptic ulcers and gastritis and protect the liver against toxins. Its antibacterial, antiviral actions help ward off a range of infections. Its diuretic action reduces fluid retention and hastens elimination of toxins.

**Cautions:** Can cause photo-sensitivity. Avoid during pregnancy and with antidepressants. Consult your practitioner before taking it if on any other medication.

## Lavandula officinalis Lavender

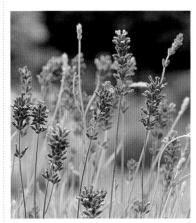

Lavender flowers calm anxiety and can relieve stress-related symptoms including muscle tension, headaches, migraines, palpitations and insomnia. Lavender lifts the spirits and dispels depression.

In the digestive system, lavender's relaxing effect eases spasm and colic and relieves wind, nausea and indigestion as well as stress-related stomach and bowel problems. It has an expectorant action and antispasmodic properties, while its antibacterial properties help fight off infections. Lavender has a mild diuretic action, making it a good cleansing remedy.

Lavender is an excellent antiseptic first aid remedy. It speeds healing by stimulating tissue repair and minimizes scar formation. When the oil is applied neat it can relieve pain and speed healing of burns and scalds, insect bites and stings, sores, wounds and ulcers.

# Leonurus cardiaca
## Motherwort

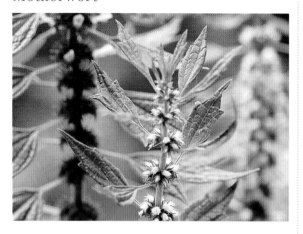

Motherwort is an interesting and attractive herb with its five-lobed leaves and whorls of pinkish flowers. It is found wild in many parts of Europe, on banks and in hedgerows. The leaves and flowers have relaxing and toning effects in the uterus. They are used for relieving period pain and regulating periods as well as for preparing for childbirth. They have a mildly sedative effect, easing tension or anxiety about the coming birth and help prevent post-partum infection and post-natal depression.

Motherwort is a good general nerve tonic, reducing anxiety, anger and irritability and menopausal mood swings as well as calming stress-related symptoms such as palpitations and irregular heart rates. It was traditionally used for strengthening and gladdening the heart and is used today for its ability to protect the heart and circulation by lowering blood pressure, reducing blood clotting and cholesterol levels.

Bitter and cooling, motherwort tea or tincture makes a good remedy for acidity and heartburn and its antispasmodic qualities can relieve stress-related digestive problems. Externally, it can be used as a douche/lotion for vaginitis and thrush.

**Caution**: Avoid using in early pregnancy. Only use a few weeks prior to the birth.

# Matricaria recutita/Anthemis nobilis/Chamaemelum nobile Chamomile

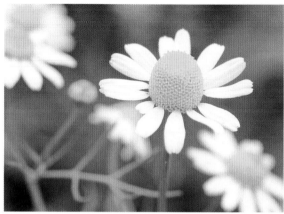

German chamomile (*Matricaria recutita*) and Roman chamomile (*Anthemis nobilis/Chamaemelum nobile*) are great for stress-related problems, particularly if they affect digestion and cause problems such as acid indigestion, peptic ulcers and wind. Chamomile is famous for calming babies, easing colic, teething and sleeping problems and for calming irritable children. Taken in tea at night it induces restful sleep. Its analgesic properties soothe discomfort and can relieve headaches, neuralgia, toothache, the aches and pains of flu, arthritis and gout. It relaxes tense muscles in the gut and helps regulate peristalsis. It can reduce symptoms of PMS, menstrual headaches and can be given for absence of periods due to stress, for mastitis and menopausal changes, to relieve nausea in pregnancy and ease contractions in childbirth. A natural antihistamine, it can relieve hay fever, allergic rhinitis, eczema and asthma. By increasing immunity, reducing inflammation, and with its antibacterial and antifungal actions, it can be used for fevers and infections. Its antiseptic and anti-inflammatory action is excellent for healing ulcers, sores, burns and scalds and skin disorders.

**Caution:** Chamomile may cause allergic reactions, including skin rash, difficulty breathing, hives, or other hypersensitivity reactions. Avoid chamomile if you are allergic to plants in the Asteraceae/Compositae family.

# Melissa officinalis
## Lemon balm

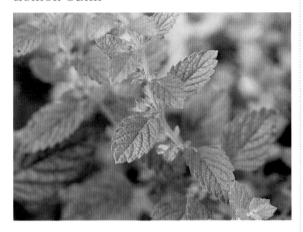

Lemon balm is a lovely lemon-scented perennial, much loved for its refreshing taste and smell. The leaves and flowers can be added to summer drinks and fruit cups, salads and desserts and make a delicious tea. Melissa is the Greek name for bee, as lemon balm is loved by bees and when planted near to bee hives it will attract new members to the colony.

Lemon balm is a wonderful remedy for the nervous system, helping to lift depression, calm anxiety, release tension, enhance relaxation and promote restful sleep. It is excellent when studying, to enhance concentration and soothe stress or exam nerves and can relieve nervous headaches and neuralgia.

It has an affinity for the digestive system, calming tension and soothing irritation and inflammation. Taken as tea or tincture, it is good for nervous indigestion, colic, wind, nausea, diarrhoea and stress related digestive disorders. It also calms the heart and relaxes spasm in the reproductive system that causes period pain. It can relieve symptoms of PMS and if taken prior to childbirth will ease the birth and lessen pain. In hot tea it reduces fevers, clears catarrhal congestion and is an excellent remedy for infections, bacterial and viral, such as herpes and mumps. It acts as an antihistamine for allergies such as hay fever and eczema.

# Mentha piperita
## Peppermint

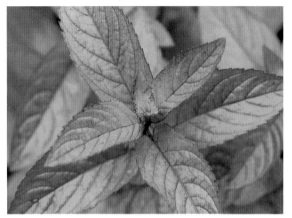

Mint makes an excellent digestive remedy, stimulating the appetite and improving digestion and absorption. It has a relaxant and anti-inflammatory effect, relieving pain and spasm in the gut and can be used for stomach aches, colic, wind, heartburn, indigestion, nausea, vomiting and travel sickness. As tea or tincture mint protects the digestive tract from irritation and infection and is excellent for bowel disorders, Crohn's disease and ulcerative colitis. It stimulates the liver and gall bladder, helping cleanse the liver and preventing gall stones developing.

Mintˆs antispasmodic action eases tension and spasm. Its analgesic properties help relieve pain, relieving headaches, migraine, back pain, sciatica, arthritis and gout. The volatile oils that give its wonderful taste and smell have effective antibacterial, antiviral, antifungal and antiparasitic properties. A hot tea is excellent when taken at the first signs of infection. Taken in a hot tea, mint disperses blood to the surface and causes sweating, making a first-rate remedy for fevers and for cleansing the body by enhancing elimination of toxins via the pores. Its astringent, decongestant action helps to relieve catarrhal congestion. When applied to the skin peppermint can clear ringworm and cold sores. As a gargle it can be used for sore throats and as a mouthwash for gum problems and mouth ulcers.

# Ocimum basilicum
## Basil

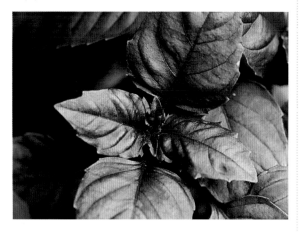

Basil is a tender annual with a lovely, pungent clove-like fragrance; a favourite in Mediterranean cuisine. It can be grown in pots on a sunny windowsill or in the garden in summer, once all danger of frost has passed. The leaves are delicious with tomatoes, in salads, soups, pasta sauces and casseroles

Basil is an excellent, relaxing nerve tonic, It makes a good natural tranquillizer, relieving tension and anxiety and lifting the spirits. At the same time it is energizing and can relieve tiredness and lethargy. It clears the mind and improves concentration and memory and makes a good remedy for stress-related symptoms including migraines, headaches, nerve pain, indigestion and muscle tension, colic as well as tight coughs, asthma and period pains. Taken hot, basil tea acts as a decongestant, so it is well worth taking for colds, flu, catarrh, catarrhal coughs and sore throats. Its antiseptic properties help fight off infections. It has a relaxing effect in the respiratory tract, useful in asthma and tight coughs and in the digestive tract, relieving cramp, diarrhoea, nausea and constipation. You can rub basil leaves on to minor cuts and grazes, bites and stings.

# Ocimum sanctum
## Tulsi, sacred basil, holy basil

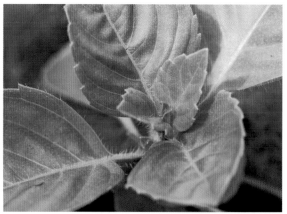

Holy basil is an excellent aid to the digestive system; it makes a delicious remedy for pain and colic, wind and bloating, and improves digestion and absorption. It acts as a laxative, is probiotic and anthelmintic and has anti-ulcer activity. It can be used in anorexia, nausea, vomiting, dysbiosis, candida and worms. Holy basil also has anti-inflammatory, immune-enhancing and adaptogenic actions, enhancing the body's resistance to stress of all kinds; it protects healthy cells from toxicity from radiation and chemotherapy and protects the heart from damage caused by chemotherapy. It lowers blood sugar, cholesterol and triglyceride levels. It has a relaxing effect on the respiratory system and acts as a decongestant, expectorant and antihistamine. It is an excellent remedy for allergies such as hay fever, rhinitis, asthma and bronchial congestion.

Holy basil is great for nerves. It is uplifting and excellent in anxiety, mild depression, insomnia and for relieving stress-related problems such as headaches and IBS. In the urinary system a lukewarm tea can relieve cystitis and urinary tract infections and clears toxins through its diuretic effect. You can apply the juice of fresh leaves to allergic skin rashes, athlete's foot and acne. Its antibiotic effect speeds healing.

**Caution:** Avoiding during pregnancy.

# Origanum marjorana
## Marjoram

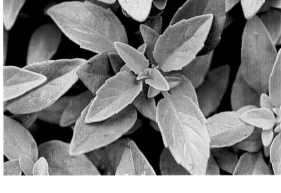

Marjoram leaves and flowers have warming and relaxing properties. They improve circulation and relieve problems such as chilblains and cramps; they release muscle tension, easing abdominal pain, menstrual cramps, headaches and aching muscles.

Marjoram tea or tincture makes a good tonic to the nerves, easing tension and anxiety, lifting the spirits, improving energy and yet inducing sleep. It is excellent for stress-related symptoms, particularly in the digestive system. It stimulates the appetite and promotes digestion and absorption and can relieve indigestion, nausea, wind, spastic colon and constipation. Its volatile oils are highly antiseptic and make marjoram a good medicine for stomach and bowel infections and for a wide range of other infections. Marjoram is well worth taking with or after antibiotics, to help re-establish a normal bacterial population of the gut, and it makes a good immune-enhancing remedy to help ward off coughs, colds, flu and fevers. Taken as a hot tea marjoram reduces fevers and acts as an effective decongestant, excellent for treating colds, coughs, bronchial and nasal congestion, sinusitis and hayfever. The antioxidants help to protect the body against ageing, while its diuretic properties help relieve fluid retention and help elimination of toxins. Added to rubbing oils marjoram may help to relieve aching muscles and painful joints.

# Petroselinum crispum
## Parsley

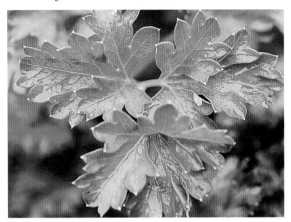

Parsley is a hardy biennial whose familiar-tasting leaves are highly nutritious. It is rich in vitamins A, B and C and minerals including iron, calcium, magnesium, manganese and sodium, as well as essential fatty acids. Parsley stimulates the appetite and improves digestion and absorption and makes a good tonic when you are run down or anaemic. Its digestive properties enable those with weak digestions to benefit from its nourishing vitamins and minerals.

Parsley has a relaxing effect, relieving colic, wind and nervous indigestion as well as headaches, migraine, asthma and irritable bladder. Its antiseptic volatile oils help combat infections. The leaves and seeds stimulate the kidneys and act as a diuretic, useful in urinary infections and fluid retention, and for clearing toxins from the body that contribute to arthritis and gout. Parsley stimulates the uterine muscles, promoting contractions during childbirth and increasing the supply of breast milk. It also stimulates the circulation and acts as a tonic to the nervous system, relieving anxiety and depression. Crushed fresh leaves can relieve irritation of insect stings. Cooked in wine and applied as a poultice they were an old remedy for bruises and sprains, as was parsley juice to relieve toothache or earache.

**Caution:** Avoid during pregnancy and kidney disease.

# Plantago major/minor/lanceolata
## Plantain

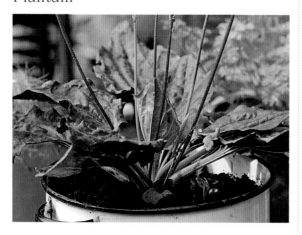

Plantain is a familiar perennial, frequently found growing in lawns, footpaths, cultivated land and waste ground, easily recognized by its cylindrical spikes of seeds. It varies from being broad leaved, to smaller leaved and *P. lanceolata* has long narrow leaves that are ribbed. The young leaves make a nutritious addition to salads.

Plantain leaves have a soothing action throughout the body, particularly in the respiratory, digestive and urinary systems, relieving irritated and inflamed conditions such as colitis, gastritis, bronchitis, harsh, irritating coughs and cystitis. They have an astringent action, stemming bleeding and encouraging healing internally and externally and are excellent for treating gastritis, diarrhoea and catarrh.

Plantain is antiseptic, cleansing and a good expectorant. A hot tea or tincture can be taken for colds, sinus congestion and allergic conditions such as hay fever and asthma. The fresh leaves can be applied to nettle, wasp and bee stings, mosquito and flea bites.

# Prunella vulgaris
## Self-heal

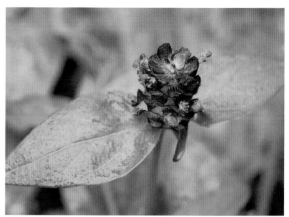

Self-heal, as the name suggests, is used to enhance our own healing powers and immunity. The leaves and flowers can be used to support the nervous system in times of stress and can help relieve headaches (particularly if they are related to anxiety), vertigo, over-sensitivity to light and high blood pressure. An effective antibiotic against a range of bacterial infections, self-heal has an affinity for the lymphatic system and can be taken for swollen glands, mumps, glandular fever and mastitis. Taken in hot tea it can reduce fevers. Its detoxifying action can help clear boils and other inflammatory skin problems and can be helpful for treating gout. A tea or tincture makes a good astringent remedy for diarrhoea and inflammatory bowel problems, such as colitis, as well as heavy periods.

Self-heal is a traditional wound remedy. You can apply the tea or the fresh plant to stop bleeding from cuts, reduce swelling from minor injuries and burns, bites and stings, and inflammatory skin problems, piles, varicose veins and ulcers. The tea or tincture makes a good astringent gargle for sore throats, a mouthwash for mouth ulcers and bleeding gums or a lotion for cooling inflammatory eye problems, including conjunctivitis, blepharitis and styes.

# Rosa spp
## Rose

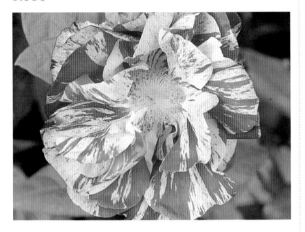

Roses act to enhance the efforts of the immune system and will help clear cold and flu symptoms, sore throats, catarrh and chest infections. In the digestive tract they help re-establish normal bacterial population when disrupted. Their astringent action reduces hyperacidity and stomach overactivity, which causes excessive hunger, thirst and mouth ulcers. Rosehip syrup or decoction of empty seed cases relieves diarrhoea, stomach cramps, constipation, nausea and indigestion. Rose petals and hips are antiseptic and diuretic; they reduce inflammation and dissolve stones and gravel. Taken in teas, tincture or powder they can be used to relieve urinary tract infections, fluid retention, and as a cleansing remedy to clear toxins and are helpful when treating arthritis.

Rosehips, petals and oil have a restoring effect on the nervous system, lifting the spirits and calming anxiety. They make a lovely remedy for insomnia, depression, irritability, anger, mental and physical fatigue. They have an affinity with the female reproductive system, relieving PMS, pelvic congestion, heavy periods, hot flushes, night sweats and mood swings. Rose water cleanses and tones skin, clears inflammation in acne, spots, boils, abscesses and sore eyes.

**Cautions:** Avoid in pregnancy.

# Rosmarinus officinalis
## Rosemary

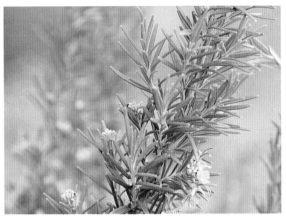

The leaves and flowers have a relaxing, stimulating effect on the central nervous system, reducing anxiety and depression while enhancing energy and concentration, mental alertness and equanimity. Rosemary is excellent for headaches and migraines, when taken on a regular basis.

Rosemary contains volatile oils, which are highly antiseptic, with antibacterial, antiviral and antifungal properties, enhancing the function of the immune system. Hot rosemary tea makes an excellent remedy for the first signs of colds, flu, coughs and chest infections and to bring down fevers. The pungent, stimulating properties have an excellent decongestant action, effective in treating catarrh, bronchial congestion, wheezing and asthma. Its warming, stimulating properties increase the flow of digestive juices and bile, improving digestion and liver function, so helping to detoxify the system. It is excellent for liver problems, gallstones, jaundice and, by cleansing the system of toxins and wastes, for gout, arthritis and skin problems. Applied to the skin, rosemary has a warming effect and by bringing blood to the surface it helps resolve inflammation and speed healing. It can be used for healing cuts and wounds, sores, chilblains, scalds and burns. It makes an excellent remedy for soothing painful arthritic joints, aching muscles and for treating local infections such as thrush.

# Salvia officinalis
## Sage

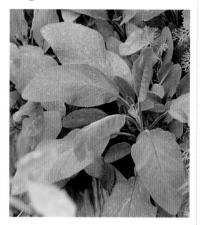

Sage is wonderful for the nerves and has a reputation as a brain tonic and longevity remedy. It is excellent for infections and can be taken for colds, flu, fevers, sore throats and chest infections. Its diuretic properties make it a good detoxifying remedy, useful for treating arthritis and gout. In the digestive tract it relaxes tension and colic, stimulates appetite and digestion and helps the liver in its detoxifying work. It protects the gut lining from irritation and inflammation and helps to relieve diarrhoea. Sage can be taken for period problems and its oestrogenic properties make it helpful for menopausal problems. It is an excellent antiseptic first-aid remedy. Use it as a gargle for sore throats, a mouthwash for inflamed gums and mouth ulcers, or a lotion or douche for vaginal infections.

**Caution:** Avoid during pregnancy and while breastfeeding.

# Salvia sclarea
## Clary sage

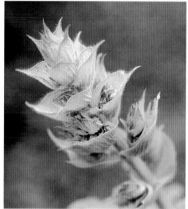

Clary sage is a lovely relaxant and nerve tonic, recommended for stress-related problems such as headaches, insomnia and indigestion. The leaves and flowers can be made into preparations for pain and spasm in the digestive system, for period pains and contractions during childbirth. It has a strengthening effect, reducing tiredness and exhaustion and lifting depression, particularly after childbirth.

Clary sage has an affinity for the respiratory system, relieving asthma and harsh irritating coughs. Similar to red sage, it is used for excessive perspiration – useful during the menopause, especially since it has oestrogenic properties. It makes a soothing lotion for the eyes.

**Caution:** Avoid during pregnancy and do not mix with alcohol.

# Scutellaria lateriflora
## Virginian skullcap

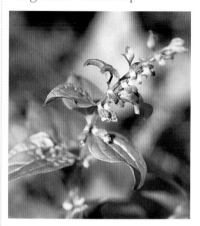

Virginian skullcap leaves and flowers are rich in nutrients, essential to a healthy nervous system and are a perfect tonic for supporting busy, stressful lives.

Skullcap relaxes and soothes the nerves, helps reduce anxiety and ease tense, aching muscles. It calms restlessness, lifts depression, dispels tiredness and when taken before bed promotes sleep. It is a great remedy when feeling nervously overwrought or run down and when wanting to stay off or withdraw from orthodox tranquillizers and antidepressants. When combined with hormone-balancing herbs such as vitex, skullcap is good for reducing emotional symptoms of PMS and the menopause and helps steady mood swings. It helps relieve pain including nervous headaches and arthritis, can be used for palpitations, epilepsy, stress-related digestive problems and when taken hot helps lower fevers.

# Stachys betonica
## Wood betony

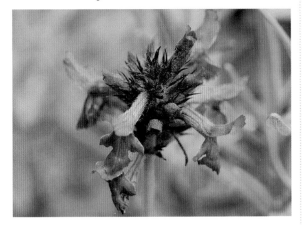

# Taraxacum officinale
## Dandelion

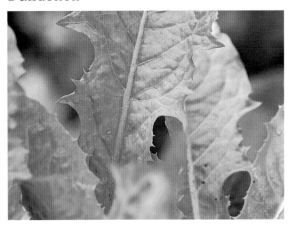

The flowers and leaves of wood betony are a great remedy for headaches from a variety of causes, including poor circulation to the head, a sluggish liver and tension. They are ideal for supporting the nervous system in times of stress. Wood betony is also excellent for soothing nerve pain such as sciatica.It is cleansing and pain-relieving for arthritis, gout and rheumatism and is traditionally used for convulsions and nervous palpitations. In the reproductive system it relieves period pain and PMS, stimulates uterine muscle and can bring on delayed periods. It is cooling and relaxing for menopausal problems.

Wood betony is a good remedy for the digestion and liver, easing indigestion, colic, wind, liver and gall-bladder problems, as well as diarrhoea. It has a decongestant action and when taken in hot tea helps to throw off head colds, catarrh, sinusitis and coughs. It also lowers blood sugar. In lotions and creams for the skin wood betony stems bleeding, speeds repair and inhibits infection of cuts and wounds, sores, ulcers, varicose veins and haemorrhoids, bruises, sprains and strains and can be used simply to beautify the skin. It will help draw splinters and thorns and is traditionally taken as snuff for nosebleeds and headaches.

**Cautions:** Avoid during pregnancy.

The young leaves are highly nutritious and can be used to add a mildly bitter touch to salads. The roasted roots make an excellent coffee substitute.

Dandelion is a bitter digestive and liver tonic, enhancing appetite and promoting digestion. The roots and leaves are gently detoxifying by their action on the liver and diuretic properties, aiding elimination of toxins via the kidneys. The young leaves are traditionally eaten in spring as a cleanser and tonic and the root is used to treat liver problems, hepatitis, gall-bladder infections, gall stones and symptoms associated with a sluggish liver such as tiredness, headaches, irritability and skin problems. Using dandelion regularly can also be helpful for arthritis, gout, fluid retention, urinary infections, prostate problems as well as for indigestion and constipation. You can apply the white juice from the stems to get rid of warts.

Dandelion's therapeutic action in the digestive tract extends to the pancreas, where it helps regulate insulin secretion and so can be useful to diabetics and hypoglycaemics.

**Caution:** The milky juice, if sucked excessively by children, can cause nausea, vomiting or diarrhoea.

# Thymus vulgaris
## Thyme

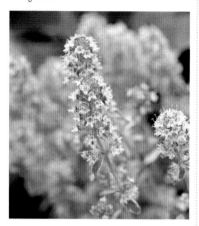

As a tea, tincture or an inhalation of the essential oil, thyme enhances immunity and helps fight infection. Its combined antimicrobial, expectorant and muscle-relaxing actions are excellent for respiratory and chest infections. In the digestive tract thyme can ease tension causing wind or indigestion. Its astringent effect protects the gut lining from irritation, inflammation and infection, while its antimicrobial action is excellent for treating gut infections.

Thyme is a good warming herb for poor circulation. It dispels mental and physical exhaustion, relieves tension and lifts depression. As a cleansing remedy it helps clear toxins via the lungs, the bowels, the skin and the urinary system. Its diuretic and antiseptic properties relieve cystitis and irritable bladder when combined with soothing herbs, and aid elimination of uric acid and toxins that contribute to gout and arthritis.

# Tropaeolum majus
## Nasturtium

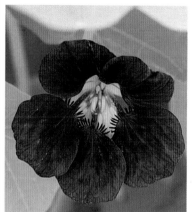

Nasturtium leaves and flowers have a bitter, pungent taste, invigorating the digestion, improving appetite and absorption and are excellent for treating weak digestion and a sluggish liver. They stimulate liver, pancreas and gall-bladder action and the secretion of digestive enzymes and ensure healthy bowel function. Nasturtium also has a diuretic action and with its antimicrobial properties, makes a good remedy for urinary infections and fluid retention. It is a good blood cleanser, improves the circulation and enhances immunity. It acts as a decongestant and is excellent for anyone feeling run down and prone to infections.

Nasturtium's main uses are as a treatment for respiratory infections. It is an expectorant as well as an antibiotic, antiseptic and antifungal.

# Urtica dioica
## Nettle

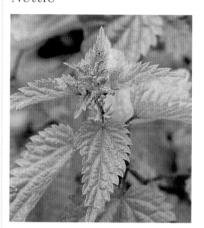

Nettles are highly nutritious, rich in vitamins and minerals, particularly iron, calcium, silica and potassium. They make a nourishing spring tonic when you are run down. By stimulating the action of the liver and kidneys they help to cleanse the body of toxins. By increasing excretion of uric acid they help to relieve gout and arthritis and reduce blood sugar. Nettle seeds help to improve thyroid function and reduce goitre, while the root is excellent for enlargement of the prostate. Nettles are a natural diuretic and can relieve fluid retention, cystitis and urethritis. Their astringent properties reduce bleeding; the fresh juice or tea can be applied to cuts and wounds to stop bleeding and speed healing. They stimulate milk production, are rich in iron, and help to increase haemoglobin levels in anaemia. Hot nettle tea helps clear catarrhal congestion and reduce fevers and makes a good remedy for allergies such as eczema and asthma.

# Verbena officinalis
## Vervain

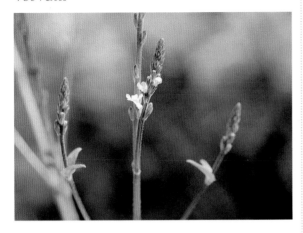

Vervain is a hardy perennial found growing wild in hedgerows and dry, barren places, with pretty but small lilac-coloured flowers on slender spikes. It is grown in France and other European countries, where vervain tea made from the leaves and flowers continues to be very popular.

Vervain is an excellent tonic to the nervous system, helping to calm the nerves, lift depression and support the body during stress. It can be thought of for most stress-related symptoms, such as headaches, indigestion, insomnia, high blood pressure, aches and pains and nervous exhaustion.

Vervain is also a good herb for the digestion, enhancing appetite and improving digestion and absorption. Its bitter taste stimulates the liver, the great detoxifying organ of the body, helping to cleanse the system and relieve symptoms such as headaches, irritability and constipation. Taken in hot tea it brings down fevers and taken cool it has a diuretic and detoxifying action and is a good remedy for cystitis. It enhances milk supply in feeding mothers and helps regulate periods.

# Viola tricolor
## Wild pansy

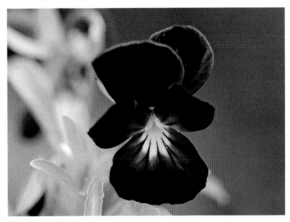

This pretty annual, with its lovely heart-shaped flowers, can be found growing wild in corn fields and cultivated ground and the plant is of great value when grown in containers as it flowers repeatedly from spring to autumn.

The leaves and flowers of wild pansy have soothing and expectorant effects, good for inflammatory chest problems, bronchitis, harsh, irritating coughs, whooping cough, asthma and croup. Taken in hot tea it relieves catarrhal congestion and brings down fevers.

Its soothing diuretic action relieves cystitis and fluid retention and has a detoxifying effect. It is often prescribed to cool the system and clear skin conditions and its salicylates are helpful for treating arthritis and gout. It has a beneficial effect on the circulation, reducing blood pressure, strengthening blood vessels and helping to prevent arteriosclerosis.

# Index

# Acknowledgements

Produced by **Bookworx**
Editor: Jo Godfrey Wood, Designer: Peggy Sadler

Publisher: Sarah Ford
Managing Editor: Camilla Davis
Photographer: Juliette Wade
Designer: Eoghan O' Brien
Senior Production Controller: Caroline Alberti

All photography by Juliette Wade except page 127 middle, Alamy/
Brad Perks Lightscapes

Thanks to Sian Hemmings for her assistance in growing the herbs
and planting the pots